TERRAIN THERAPY

TERRAIN THERAPY

How To Achieve **Perfect Health** Through
Diet, Living Habits & Divine Thinking

from the wisdom of
DR. ULRIC WILLIAMS

with foreword and updates by
Dr. Samantha Bailey

Copyright © 2022 by Samantha Bailey
www.drsambailey.com
All rights reserved

Terrain Therapy: How To Achieve Perfect Health Through Diet, Living Habits & Divine Thinking
Based on: Hints on Healthy Living (original title)
First published in 1934 by Wanganui Chronicle Print, New Zealand

Paperback ISBN: 978-1-99-118550-1
Hardcover ISBN: 978-1-99-118551-8
Ebook ISBN: 978-1-99-118552-5

DISCLAIMER

The information contained herein should NOT be used as a substitute for the advice of an appropriately qualified health care provider. The information and content provided here are for informational purposes only. In the event you use any of the information in this book for yourself or your dependents, you assume full responsibility for your actions.

"As a man thinketh in his heart, so is he."

            Proverbs XXIII, 7.

"The man that closes his mind to that which is strange or new is afraid — he dislikes untrodden paths."

            Dr. Ulric Williams

Contents

Foreword by Dr Samantha Bailey 13

Foreword to First and Second Editions 22

Foreword to Third Edition 24

Introduction to Fourth Edition...27

Foreword to Fifth Edition 39

1. What Disease is, and How it is Brought About......................45
    Man's Dwelling Place..46
    Sins of Commission..47
    Symptoms – Their Dual Significance............................47
    Costly Blundering...48
    Not Interested...49
    Then and Now...49
    Defective Polarization..50

2. Disease Defined; The Cause of Disease 51
    The Primary Causes 51
    The Secondary Causes 53
    Mineral Deficiency...57
    Toxic Accumulation..59
    "Fifteen Points" of Pollution..60
    The Calcium Thieves..62

3. Orthodox Medical Methods Cause Disease 64
    Orthodox Methods Never "Cure" Disease....................65
    Symptoms and Diagnosis...66

    The Invariable Mistake. 68

    Familiar Suppressive Measures. 68

    Vaccines and Sera...71

    Surgical Operations. 73

    The Tonsil and Appendix Racket. 75

    The Cancer Industry: Radium, X-rays, and Cancer Research. 76

    Hospital Folly. 78

    Mental Disease. 79

    The Last Straw. 80

    Misaligned Systems...81

    Orthodox Opposition. 82

4. **The Problem of Treatment — General Considerations** 83

    I. The Dawn of a Better Day 83

    Relief, or Reform. 84

    A Purpose in Suffering. 85

    Only One Way. 85

    II. Right Thinking 86

    Spiritual Physics..87

    "Jacob's Trouble." 88

    Creative Power. 89

    Penalties Exacted by Misuse. 90

    Thoughts are Vibratory Forces...91

    What We Think and Speak of, We Bring into Being. 91

    Consider the Lillies..93

5. **The Part Man Must Play**...95

6. **Correcting Psychological Causes**..97

    I. Wrong Mental and Emotional Thoughts........................97

Don't Fight Disease, but Practice Good Health.................98
Gland Influence and Control. 98
Some Effects of Disturbance...................................99
The Valley of Decision...101
"I Will Bring Evil . . ."..101
"Quietness and Confidence Shall be Thy Strength."..........103
"The Kingdom of Good is Within." 104
"Thou Wilt Keep Him in Perfect Peace Whose Mind is Stayed on Thee."...105
Practise the Presence of God. 106
"Perfect Love Casteth out Fear." 106
II. Wrong Ideas in the Subconscious Mind.................107
The Subconscious Trap. 108

7. Correcting Physical Causes 112
I. Misuse of foods 112
Commonsense Foods, not "Diet." 112
The Food Ramp. 113
Scatty Indifference. 114
The "Ape's" Final Fling. 114
Refined Foods are Dead Foods; and Dead Foods are Death-Dealing..115
Suicidal Imbecility..115
The Real Cause of Poliomyelitis. 120
Why Spoil our Foods? 123
Protective Foods..123
In Conclusion. 126
One Final Word. 127
II. Faulty General Habits....................................127
III. Supply Deficiencies and Promote Elimination 132

- Promoting Elimination. 133
- **IV. Correcting Secondary Causes** **135**
- Mechanical. 135
- Economic. 136

8. Helping Nature Cure 138
- **I. The Healing Crises** **138**
- The Gospel of "Nature Cure." 139
- These are Nature's Healing Crises. 140
- Nature's Efforts to Cure. Their Onset, and Action. 141
- Duration. 142
- The Periodicity of Disease. 143
- Parenthetically. 144
- Procedure. 144
- **II. The Part Played by Fasting** **145**
- Caution. 146
- Duration of a Fast. 147
- Phenomena Commonly Observed During a Fast. 149

9. Mental And Spiritual Healing 151
- **I. Faith Healing.** **151**
- "Can God?" 155
- **II. How Faith Works** **156**
- Vital Considerations. 157
- "Greater Things than These." 159
- Power Unlimited. 160
- The Justification for Faith. 161
- "Christ in You, the Hope of Glory." 161
- **III. Higher Healing Resources** **163**
- Absent Treatment. 164

    Prayer. 165

    Mediation. 168

    IV. Divine Healing **169**

    Spiritual Subterfuge. 169

    The Real Objective. 170

10. Illustrative Examples **172**

11. The Healing Spirit Made Manifest **181**

12. The Standard Diet **185**

    Rules of Eating. 185

    Breakfast. 186

    Lunch. 187

    Suggestions for Workingmen's Lunches and Picnics. 188

    Dinner. 189

    Suggested Diet for One Week. 190

13. Dietary Principles For Children **194**

    Weaning the Infant. 198

    Diet for child aged from 9 to 12 months. 198

    From 15 to 18 months. 200

    From 18 months to 2 years. 200

    From 2 to 3½ years. 201

    Diet from 3½ to 4½ years. 203

    Diet from 4½ to 5 years. 206

    From 5½ to 7 years. 209

14. Fasting; Eliminative and Special Diets **211**

    Types of Eliminative and Special Diets 212

15. Directions For Carrying Out A Fast **213**

For Acute Illness.	213
For Chronic Disease	214

16. Eliminative and Special Diets 215
    1. Fruit Diet. 215
    2. Fruit and Vegetable Diet. 215
    3. Milk Diet. 215
    4. Eliminating Diet. 216
    5. Reducing Diet. 218
    6. Digestive Diet. 219
    7. Readjusting Diet 220
    8. Heavy Duty Diet. 223

17. Breaking The Fast 228

18. Suggestions For Hotel Diet 231

19. Hints on Preparation and Cooking 233
    Sweetening Fruit 235
    Measurement Conversion Table 236

Recipes Index 237

About the Authors 373

Foreword by Dr Samantha Bailey

I first discovered Dr Ulric Williams (1890-1971) in 2021. A dear friend, Simin Williams, (whose husband is distantly related to Dr Williams,) sent me a copy of *New Zealand's Greatest Doctor – Ulric Williams of Wanganui – a Surgeon who became a Naturopath.*

The booklet was published in 1998 by Brenda Sampson, who had been a former patient of Dr Williams in the 1940s. Simin met the 83-year-old Brenda in 2000 and described her as, "a picture of health, so bright eyed and sharp in mind...a tall and beautiful lady and very straight up, both physically and in her manner." However, Brenda never mentioned her publication during that meeting and it was not until several years later that Simin came across a copy of *New Zealand's Greatest Doctor* and made the connection.

The book instantly struck a chord with me on a number of levels. The first was how concise Dr Williams was with his explanations of health and disease. For example, he would say, "all disease comes from one of two places, either an unhealthy way of life...or else it comes from unhappiness in the mind and spirit."

This was in striking contrast to my allopathic medical training where I was bombarded with the names of hundreds of diseases, many of which appeared to be able to strike unsuspecting victims at will. For most of these disease entities the allopathic system postulates a single cause and a specific treatment protocol. Dr Williams saw the folly of treating people this way: there are no specific 'entities' as such, there are only the manifested symptoms and *conditions* of the body. He did not believe in 'Germ theory' and Louis Pasteur's claims; instead Dr Williams lent his support to the 'Terrain' theorist Antoine

Béchamp and stated, "it isn't the germs that matter but that upon which they prey."

Dr Williams placed a great deal of importance on the psychological and spiritual realms—he was clear that a healthy body was ultimately dependent on a healthy mind and a resolute connection on the spiritual plain. Deficiencies in this department were not only detrimental to health but sometimes fatal. As he would explain, "if a person is very unhappy and can't find a way out of the unhappiness, the body will create a way out through illness."

Dr Williams had no hubris when it came to the abilities of doctors and once said to Brenda Sampson, "I didn't cure you, only God can heal. Actually what I did, was to teach you how to cure yourself and that will be useful to you all your life."

He had not always been that way. Earlier in his career the dashing obstetrician/surgeon had a reputation of being a playboy doctor, more interested in sports, women and booze than his patients. As one friend put it, he would, "rush them through the surgery, filling them up with sedatives and drugs just as quickly as he could, so that he might have more time for his pleasures." However, Dr Williams reached a crisis point in 1931 and became horrified with the allopathic "remedies" that he had been dispensing for material profits. (He also described this turning point in the Foreword to Fifth Edition.)

He knew it was time to find a new path and over the next few years, gradually worked out his basis for healthy living—right eating, right thinking and right living with an appreciation of the relationship between body, mind and spirit. He became appalled at the number of operations being done and resolved to do no more surgery. He made detailed studies on the processing of food, the health and methods of fertilisation of the soil, diet and psychology. He concluded that the excessive use of chemical pesticides and fertilisers were endangering human health. In this regard he was years ahead of even Rachel Carson who blew the whistle on DDT and other environmental chemical contaminants in the 1960s.

In *New Zealand's Greatest Doctor,* Brenda Sampson mentioned some of Dr Williams' publications but they had all been out of print for many years. After an extensive search I managed to purchase a 1939 4th edition of *Hints on Healthy Living* from a Wellington bookshop. The book was another great revelation and I was unable to put it down. His sentences can appear simple and yet they are often powerful aphorisms — for example, "don't fight disease, but practice good health," is one of my guiding principles.

Dr Williams published the 83-page first edition of *Hints on Healthy Living* in 1934. By the 4th edition, the one I hold, it had reached 300 pages with well over 100 of the pages comprising recipes. There was a 5th edition of the book in 1949, which came with the new title *Health and Healing in the New Age.* A copy of this can be found in The National Library of New Zealand. It can get confusing when book titles are changed in this way but it was probably more fitting than a title that suggested it contained merely "hints." Although Dr Williams had humbly written in the 1930s that, "the scope of this book is indicated in its title," it is certainly instructive enough to provide the reader with a comprehensive way of living and a profound understanding of health.

When we decided to put this book into print, consideration was given as to whether to modernise the format and style. Dr Williams favoured a great deal of capitalisation in his writing which may seem unusual in the present day as he appears to be shouting at his readers. However, on reflection we elected to maintain his literary style. If he was concerned about unhealthy lifestyles in the 1930s it is almost certain that he would be shouting at us even more loudly in the 2020s. There is also a personal delight in allowing a buried voice to have a platform over 80 years later. By leaving the style as it was, Dr Williams gets to speak again in his unique style while his detractors are long since forgotten. The truth has a habit of surfacing even if it takes time.

While preserving most of his original content there have been some updates to help the modern reader. Some of Dr Williams' classifications and lists have been reorganised to make them clearer. Where more accurate and important information is now available, it has been added. What is most remarkable is how little needed changing, such is his timeless wisdom. His examples of 1930s medical follies have been left in place as they are illustrative of many of the same erroneous "health" models that are still blindly followed today. The laws of God and the nature of biology cannot be changed by man. Dr Williams' genius was in the distillation and communication of these principles to others.

There are a large number of recipes in this book, which is appropriate given the emphasis that Dr Williams placed on achieving health through diet. They are simple to follow, nourishing, and practical with the vital themes being readily apparent. Our diets should consist of foods that are provided by nature with the avoidance of processes that deplete their nutritional value. By simply browsing through the recipes you will see plenty of fruits and vegetables and unadulterated ingredients. It goes without saying that knowing where your food comes from is of the upmost importance.

Dr Williams was not averse to meat in the diet although he would advise restricting its consumption during times of illness. There are no meat dishes amongst the recipes apart from the unexpected appearance of a one 'Savoury Rabbit' in the 'Meat Substitute' section! (Our family consumes meat regularly and I am happy to leave others to work out their best balance.) Raw milk and butter, however, are frequently employed in the recipes. If flour is being used, it should usually be wholemeal, while sweetening is achieved through raw sugar or honey. Puddings can be part of a healthy diet if they consist of such wholesome ingredients. One of my favourite recipes in this book is Welsh Nectar — a natural homemade soft drink with a delicious mouthfeel that cannot be replicated by commercial varieties.

For readers outside the United Kingdom and Australasia there may be a few unfamiliar terms. *Marmite* and *Vegemite* are potent food spreads made from yeast extract. They are jet black in colour and rich sources of vitamin B compounds. *Weet-bix* is a popular breakfast cereal in Australasia, with a similar product in the UK and North America being *Weetabix*. Granose flakes are now known as Corn flakes, so this was updated in the recipes section. There are a few other 'old' words that have been preserved to remind us of our heritage. Recipe measurements are mostly in the imperial system and brief on instructions — the idea is more about appreciating the principle of natural ingredients and eating minimally manipulated food.

During his practicing career, Dr Williams gave many popular public lectures and wrote to newspapers frequently. He campaigned against fluoridation of water supplies and was opposed to all vaccines — which he described as, "disgusting and disease-producing." Such positions brought him into conflict with the British Medical Association who expelled him as a member in 1936. Subsequently, a similarly outraged Medical Council failed in their attempts to have him struck off the register in the 1940s. This resonated with me due to the Medical Council's attempts to silence me after I went public in 2020 with regard to the COVID-19 fraud. However, unlike Dr Williams, I had no desire to remain practicing within the medical system once I understood its nature.

Last century Dr Williams wrote that, "the modern medical system, to the extent of perhaps 80%, is nothing but a gigantic, cruel, ludicrous, lucrative, transparent fraud." In my view, nothing has changed except perhaps that 80% is now an underestimate of the fraud taking place. In the same article he went on to state that:

> "Doctors do not know what disease is, nor how it is brought about…Doctors, completely unaware of their significance or purpose, are taught that acute illnesses are acute diseases, which they must prevent or cure. With this object they employ a battery of destructive agents, notoriously more dangerous than the ills they are supposed to cure. Poisonous drugs, vaccines, radiation and mutilating surgery are their weapons. Perhaps the worst crime of modern medical, so-called science is the increasingly effective suppression of acute illnesses. Usually, successful suppression has one of four consequences.
> 1. The sufferer is killed.
> 2. A foundation is laid for chronic and often incurable disease.
> 3. Nature (if she can) will after period intervals, stage more of these would-be spring cleanings or Healing

Crises.

4. Nature may effect a cure in spite of treatment, in which case the doctor will claim and probably get full credit for recovery."

While it may seem a harsh critique of our profession, I have come to realise the truth of it. When Dr Barbara Starfield revealed in 2000 that around 225,000 patients were dying annually in US hospitals due to medical errors, it should have been one of the scandals of the century. Keeping in mind that this does not include the iatrogenic deaths (and injuries) happening outside the hospitals, it is clear that the medico-pharmaceutical industry has blood all over its hands. It is indeed only a medical system, not a health system.

Dr Williams felt that governments had a role in promoting the health of the population and in his introduction to the 4th edition of *Hints on Healthy Living* he provides a list of, "What Governments Should Do." I suspect that if he was alive today he may have lost faith in the notion of governments having *any* positive function in the health and well-being of the average person.

Dr Williams' insights into the wider picture were remarkable for his time. He condemned the debt-based financial system and was under no illusion as to who ultimately pulled the strings when he stated, "whosoever controls credit controls most else, it is most vitally urgent that the people as a whole should co-operate to govern themselves." And ultimately, he said, it was individuals who would determine what the ruling class did with them:

"We ourselves are to blame. Give the average man a crust

and a corner of blanket, and he's satisfied. 'It is not because tyrants oppress them that the people are slaves,' said a sage, 'it is because they are so abject that the powerful and unprincipled will inevitably exploit them.'"

As his biographer Bruce Hamilton said in 1998: "Ulric Williams was an original thinker and a forceful personality and controversialist. Although regarded by many as a crank and fanatic, in his advocacy of a healthy natural way of living, methods of treatment, scepticism about unnecessary surgery, and promotion of a diet of natural foods, he was perhaps ahead of his time." I would propose that Dr Williams' advocacy is, in fact, timeless. He was informing us that if we simply respect the laws of nature and the laws of God, then health and prosperity will follow.

At times in this book it may seem that Dr Williams is preaching in a puritanical fashion. However, he was not a supporter of organised religion in general, writing in one article that, "doctors are 'disease-mongers' and churches 'sin-factories'." And although in this book the word 'God' appears over 100 times, he was well aware of how easily this could be misinterpreted. That being so, he was known to say,

> "people have so many misconceptions about this word that it is a barrier to communication. I try instead to use the words *life* and *the life force*. Life will bring you everything good, as long as you trust it."

It is a realisation that we have everything we need and will be blessed when we place our trust in ourselves and our faith in the Divine.

Hints on Healthy Living brought so much wonderful wisdom to my family and now with my best wishes I hope to pass Dr Williams' wisdom on to you with this rekindled version called *Terrain Therapy*.

Dr. Samantha Annabel Hope Bailey, MB CHB
Christchurch, New Zealand, November 2022.

REFERENCES

Hamilton, Bruce, "Story: Williams, Ulric Gaster," *Dictionary of New Zealand Biography*, 1998.

Sampson, Brenda, *New Zealand's Greatest Doctor – Ulric Williams of Wanganui – a Surgeon who became a Naturopath*, Zealand Publishing House, 1998.

Starfield, Barbara, "Is US Health Really the Best in the World?," *JAMA*, 26 Jul 2000.

Foreword to First and Second Editions
Hints on Healthy Living
(1st ed. 1934)

IT can no longer be denied that the GREAT cause of sickness is disobedience to natural law—wrong manner of living. A very large proportion of disease from which mankind suffers is IMMEDIATELY PREVENTABLE. There is nothing arbitrary or accidental about the incidence of disease. We are sick simply in proportion to the extent of infringement of natural law. Sickness is a natural consequence of disobedience. We are excused by ignorance or incredulity no more than by neglect. Turn from wrong habits of living, comply with the law, and the consequences of deflection tend to disappear.

Adopt healthy habits in regard to exercise, sunlight and fresh air; proper rest and clothing; daily cold bath and deep breathing; instead of cooked and denatured foods in excessive quantity, rely as far as possible on a moderate amount of raw foods in the natural state, and you will find that not only is health maintained at a high level of excellence, with immunity from infection, but that, when this regime is combined with suitable periods of fasting, most of the disorders which were formerly believed to be incurable or amenable only to surgery, will be found to disappear.

The choice is left in the hands of the individual; there will be no coercion; but those who obey, automatically receive their reward. Some degree of self-denial and self-control is vitally necessary; the peace that comes only of a quiet mind is indispensable; and if it be found that these essentials result only from spiritual harmony, then such finding serves but to confirm the statement that the ultimate cause of almost all disease is error or sin—disobedience to the law of God. "The wages of sin is death." (Romans VI, 23.) Many would have it otherwise, and almost superhuman are the efforts being made to discover a means whereby man may enjoy health, happiness, prosperity and immunity from disease, the fruits of harmony with the Spirit of God, while continuing to violate every one of His commands.

When the rules of health relating to right thinking, exercise, rest, sunlight and fresh air have been complied with, we must familiarise ourselves, if we are to escape the consequences of error, with those relating to diet.

Broadly speaking, besides intemperance in eating and drinking, and indulgence in extraneous poisons such as drugs, tobacco, and alcohol, our fault lies chiefly in overindulgence in meat, refined starch and sugar; and in insufficient use of fresh fruits and vegetables. A system of diet which provides a remedy for these defects will consist, in the order of their importance, of the following foodstuffs; fruits of all varieties, some dried but mostly fresh; vegetables, as many of them as possible uncooked; dairy products; and cereals, which must be unrefined. It is the object of this booklet to outline a method whereby such a system may be effectively carried out.

Foreword to Third Edition
Hints on Healthy Living
(1936)

"But if our gospel be hid, it is hid to them that are perishing; in whom the god of this world (human physical wisdom) hath blinded the minds of them that are perishing, lest the light of the glorious gospel of Christ (the indwelling Life Spirit), who is the image of God, should shine unto them."

2 Corinthians IV, 3 & 4.

WHAT appears in this little book is written not with the object of reviling men whose skill, devotion, and high ethical standard are too well recognized to need further comment; but in the spirit of love to draw the attention, of those who are big enough to take advantage of it, to the reason for the failure of many of our efforts; to indicate a line upon which investigation may usefully proceed; and to outline a principle the practice of which has already provided a happy issue out of many afflictions.

That the orthodox healing system has fallen woefully short must surely be apparent to anyone who considers for a moment the numerous and prosperous private hospitals and homes, the increasing expense upon sanatoria, the great and growing hospital population, the teeming asylums and gaols, and the rising insanity rate; and realises that these represent but a fraction of all the suffering in the land. But the extent of the failure is even yet not understood. A searching and ruthless indictment of mistaken belief and misaligned methods is overdue, and has begun, and will continue. In contributing to this exposure, let it be SUPERABUNDANTLY CLEAR that the indictment cannot be held to apply to those who still honestly subscribe to these beliefs. Defective methods, not men, stand arraigned.

The orthodox healing system has failed for reasons that can easily be defined, and might, and ultimately will, as easily be corrected. We have failed because from our too narrow and materialistic outlook we have conceived of disease as something attacking us from without, due to germs; whereas disease whether of body, mind, soul, or estate, is mostly a gradual degenerative process going on within, due to failure to comply with the requirements of well-being. We fail because in the zones of physical limit we look outside ourselves for cause and cure of troubles arising within. We have failed because the whole complicated system of orthodox modern diagnosis and treatment is based upon a misconception that mistakes the symptom for the disease; and tinkering with effects while the cause is ignored and allowed to continue always has been and always will be followed by deplorable consequences.

Medical men are neither fools nor rogues. Like Mahomet, or Buddha, or the African witch-doctor, they interpret the Spirit of God according to their measure of understanding; but like these others, are subject to the limitations of that measure. Man has advanced thus far in his long pilgrimage towards higher consciousness through the operation of the Law, of whose functioning for the most part he has been completely unaware; but further progress will be found possible only through increasing response to the Spirit, of whom the Law is a relative expression.

A thousand of the world's greatest specialists could not hope to cover the ground now traversed by orthodoxy; and their investigation is daily becoming more intricate and involved; the pity of it being that much of our boasted knowledge is not merely useless, but, being built upon a wrong foundation, almost infinitely worse than useless; having become, indeed, the second in importance of the two great causes of disease. And so we are confronted with the position that medical men of the highest integrity, actuated often by the loftiest ideals, have been and are being, though unwittingly, responsible for greater suffering by far than they have ever been able to relieve.

A REMARKABLE PARADOX

The explanation of which is that WE HAVE TRIED TO SOLVE THE PROBLEM OF HUMAN SUFFERING FROM THE LIMITED RESOURCES OF HUMAN PHYSICAL WISDOM, WITHOUT SUFFICIENT REFERENCE TO THE SPIRIT AND LAW OF GOD.

"Know ye not that ye are the temple of God, and that the Spirit of God dwelleth in you? If any man defile the temple of God, him shall God destroy; for the temple of God is holy, which temple ye are. Let no man deceive himself. If any man among you seemeth to be wise in this world, let him become a fool, that he may be wise. For the wisdom of this world is foolishness with God. For it is written, He taketh the (worldly) wise in their own craftiness. And again, The Lord knoweth the thoughts of the wise, that they are vain."

1 Corinthians III, 16 to 20.

Introduction to Fourth Edition
Hints on Healthy Living
(1939)

"He that is not with ME is against ME; and he that gathereth not with ME scattereth abroad."

Matthew XII, 30.

DISEASE is not some mysterious inscrutable entity that attacks healthy people. Those who live healthily seldom become sick. Disease is mostly a fairly obvious consequence of failure to live healthily. We make ourselves ill.

Good health is man's birthright. Yet disease is widespread. People in the street may, to the casual observer, seem passably well. But enter their homes, and look close! There are millions and millions who ought to be happy and well, pining through long years of avoidable, often easily correctable, suffering and decay; children born under the dark shadow of disease and premature death; wretched sufferers subjected, at constantly recurring ruinous expense, to repeated suppressions of Nature's patient efforts to heal—quite simple difficulties being, habitually, complicated and intensified until fear, dejection, hopelessness, and heart-breaking pain wear a weary course to tragic conclusion.

WAKE UP YOU PEOPLE!

There are going to be some heart-searchings when the public perceives the enormities that have been and are being perpetrated in the name of surgery and medicine; avoidable, mutilating, and futile operations, disgusting and disease-producing vaccines and sera, expensive and deadly drugs, which often fail even to modify symptoms, and certainly never, under any circumstances, have any beneficial effect upon causes; while Nature—God, through His natural law—has made provision, in perfect and merciful simplicity, for both prevention and cure.

Self-confident, credulous man, deluded by worship of physical wisdom, is blind to the truth.

Worship God in Spirit and in Truth; fill the mind with positive thoughts; eat Nature's foods in accordance only with need; obey the commonsense rules with regard to exercise and rest, sunlight and fresh air (to the skin, not merely to the outside of clothing), breathing, water, clothing, and posture; and disease, which is mostly a result of failure to comply with these requirements, will rapidly disappear.

THIS BUSINESS OF DISEASE.

The Business of Disease has become the second largest in the world today, the greatest being the Financial Business, with which, like the Armament Industry, it is intimately bound up. Capital to the extent of millions, and tens and hundreds of millions, is invested in the Disease Business; and the object is— PROFIT. Let the down-trodden, deluded victims reflect: *who provides the bulk of this capital, and who reaps the increase?*

One thing is certain: all that "money" will hardly be thrown away! No one can set the people free but the people themselves; and the price of liberation is absolute submission—to the Divine Spirit whose service is perfect freedom.

The people are being decimated, in a large measure due to ignorance, by easily preventable and often easily curable poverty and disease; and those who could enlighten them are carefully kept away.

Those who are making a good thing out of the people's miseries control practically all the avenues of publicity; and by their direction, press, radio, and picture screen are grinding out at high pressure misleading and lying medical and financial propaganda.

This diabolical obstructiveness is authenticated and approved not merely by powerful selfish interests, but also, though mostly unwittingly, by civic authorities, politicians, economists, hospital and asylum boards, educational powers, ministers of religion, Government and Department of Health, by manufacturers, vendors, advertisers, and consumers of death-dealing rubbish, and so ultimately and individually by the benighted sufferers themselves.

And so the public agonies are traded upon with a comprehensiveness the more exasperating because largely unconscious; and thousands of sufferers still wend their weary and ruinous way from hospital to hospital, from one orthodox medical man to another, from one futile expedient to the next

<u>AND NONE OF THEM IS EVER CURED.</u>

Our aim as communities of individuals should be, as with the communities of cells composing our bodies, to associate to mutual advantage. But, individually or collectively, we can govern ourselves successfully ONLY TO THE DEGREE OF RESPONSE TO DIVINE SPIRIT AND LAW.

Governments must be servants, not masters—representatives elected to carry into effect the spiritually aligned will of the people.

Theocracy, via democracy, is the ONLY way; NOT, as in all countries today, dictatorships—either overt as in the totalitarian states, or covert as in the misnamed democracies "where the choice lies between being hung drawn and quartered or boiled in oil."

WARNING.

The gravest possible menace threatens countries where control of credit is abused. Even when a "Government"—that is to say, the representatives of a political party—have taken control, it by no means follows that credit will be administered to the greatest advantage. For example, a *Government may be dominated by the most powerful and militant section of its supporters.* Which is equivalent to saying, by the most ruthless and dominant individuals in that section.

Since it is an axiom that whosoever controls credit controls most else, it is most *vitally urgent* that the people as a whole should co-operate to govern themselves. Otherwise, it is a certainty that they will be dictated to. The issue lies between spiritual freedom on the one hand, and materialistic capitalism or materialistic communism on the other.

Nimrod set out to build, by physical means, a tower that should reach to heaven; but confusion fell upon his followers. In Babylon, a mighty material empire held sway. But the writing appeared on the wall; and not one trace has survived. Upon the banners of both these great powers appeared the identical device:

a hammer, a sickle, and a sheaf of wheat—symbols of *human* resource and achievement.

In other countries today, similar attempts are being made—the same Devil, today as ever (human physical wisdom), deluding man with belief in his own ability to achieve, divorced from Divine Spirit and Law. And so in the mass, as in the individual, the struggle resolves itself into a conflict between the higher spiritual and lower physical of Adamic duality.

With "National Health Insurance Schemes" imminent or in force in so many countries, it were well to examine the position in principle, for obviously schemes badly at fault in principle can hardly be expected to produce the best of results, applied.

In order correctly to assess its probable effectiveness, any proposal, undertaking, or plan, will have to be subjected to three crucial tests:—

1. Is the proposal right in Spirit?
2. Is it adequate in Functioning?
3. Does it measure up in Science?

If the proposal can be shown to fall far short under any of these three headings, positive results CANNOT BE ACHIEVED. (L. E. Bassett.)

Applying these tests to the New Zealand Government's 1938-1939 proposals for "National Health Insurance," the proposals are immediately disclosed to be

VERY GRAVELY DEFECTIVE IN SCIENCE.

1. In Spirit, the proposals are right enough. Few question the Government's sincere desire to improve the health of the people, and make better provision for dealing with disease.
2. In Functioning, the proposals are adequate. Everyone acknowledges and admires the Government's energy and enthusiasm in prosecuting its objectives.

3. IN SCIENCE, THE PROPOSALS ARE DANGEROUSLY ADRIFT, because:

   (a) They assume orthodox medical methods to be curative; whereas applying the same three tests, orthodox medical methods are at once seen to be (in Spirit, often, as well as in Science), so gravely deficient as to be actually and actively causative.

   (b) They have the effect of enslaving the people more helplessly than ever to the second of the two great conscienceless monopolies (the financial being the first) from which it should be the Government's first duty to protect them.

   (c) The method of financing them is CONTRARY TO ECONOMIC PRINCIPLE. Further to reduce, by avoidable taxation, the already heavily depleted purchasing power of the steadily diminishing productive section of the people, in order to supply an always increasing non-productive section with their rightful share of goods and services available in superabundance, is not merely oppressive and unjustifiable—it is just plain stupid. "It is tantamount to pumping the sap from the trunk of a sick tree, and spraying it on to the shrivelling branches." (L. E. B.)

   > After all, since we can produce much more of the essentials of life than we are able to consume,
   >
   > WHY NOT GIVE THEM THEIR SHARE?
   >
   > How?—By giving them the requisite tickets.

   (d) Provision is not limited to those genuinely prevented from providing for themselves. Instead, sickness and endless expensive and disease-producing "treatment" are made attractive, as well as accessible, to very large numbers who refuse to make any attempt to live healthily. The "Father" (Spirit) "in dealing with the prodigal son did NOT, as the Government proposes to do, go down to the pig-stye with blankets and hot water bottles." He awaited the culprit's repentance and reform before He met him partway.

(e) They are NEGATIVE; they deal with Disease, not with Health.

(f) They IMPOSE a fallacious political theory; whereas the object can be quickly (and cheaply) attained BY CONFORMING TO DIVINE SPIRIT AND LAW.

(g) NEITHER DISEASE NOR ECONOMIC MALFUNCTIONING CAN BE CURED BY DEALING WITH SYMPTOMS. Unless they look deep enough, Governments, exactly as do orthodox medical men, mistake the symptom for the disease; and so confine their efforts to dealing with effects, while the true causes—always ultimately spiritual—are ignored and allowed to continue. And tinkering with effects while causes continue is exactly why a smiling land uniquely equipped for well-being is littered and plastered with the sick, the halt, and the dead.

WHAT GOVERNMENTS SHOULD DO.

Governments' first concern should be—NOT to fight disease—but to INCULCATE HEALTH, and FIGHT THE CAUSES OF DISEASE. To which end they should ENABLE, TEACH, and ENCOURAGE THE PEOPLE to live healthily.

In pursuing this object it is useless looking to orthodoxy for help. In finance, as in medicine, education, and religion, the relentless and uncompromising opposition of orthodoxy to reform will have to be reckoned upon.

In addition, the stranglehold of powerful interests operating in many fields must be openly and decisively challenged, *not propitiated*; and the people's support mobilised to make the challenge effective.

A SICK MAN RECOVERS RAPIDLY. IN MOST CASES, WHEN THE CAUSES OF HIS MISFORTUNES ARE CORRECTED.

But many eager to know how to do this are being deliberately and systematically misled.

TO MAKE EFFECTIVE PROVISION FOR HEALTH,
Governments must:

1. OPENLY ACKNOWLEDGE GOD AS LEADER AND HEAD; AND DO THEIR UTMOST TO LEARN AND CONFORM TO HIS WAY, WHICH IS COMPLETE AND READY TO HAND.

2. INTENSIVELY EDUCATE PARENTS, BY EVERY AVAILABLE CHANNEL, IN NATURAL AND SPIRITUAL METHODS BOTH OF PREVENTION AND TREATMENT.

3. EDUCATE THE CHILDREN, FROM EARLIEST SCHOOL AGE, IN THE SCIENCE OF RIGHT THINKING AND HEALTHY LIVING.

4. HAVING TAKEN FULL CONTROL OF CREDIT AND CURRENCY, DO THEIR UTMOST, IN CONTINUAL COOPERATION WITH THE PEOPLE, TO SEE THAT ADMINISTRATION IS IN HARMONY WITH DIVINE SPIRIT AND LAW.

5. SEE THAT ENOUGH DEFENSIVE FOODS (FRUITS, VEGETABLES, DAIRY PRODUCTS, AND WHOLE GRAINS) OF HIGHEST QUALITY ONLY, ARE AVAILABLE FREE, OR AT THE CHEAPEST RATE, TO ALL.
6. ABOLISH ALL FOOD REFINING AND ADULTERATION; AND SET UP MACHINERY FOR DETERMINING FOOD VALUES AND PUBLISHING THEM.
7. ABOLISH ALL HARMFUL DRUGS.
8. DEAL COSMICALLY (!) WITH HUMUS AND MINERAL DEFICIENCY IN PASTURES, ORCHARDS AND GARDENS.
9. PROVIDE FOR SCIENTIFIC SEWAGE DISPOSAL; AND PLANTING AND CARE OF FORESTS. (Stone.)
10. CENSOR ADVERTISEMENTS.
11. IMMEDIATELY INCREASE, WITHOUT INCREASING TAXATION, FAMILY ALLOWANCE AND PENSIONS; AND MAKE SUPERVISED PROVISION FOR SICKNESS AND ACCIDENT.
12. PENSION OFF THE LARGE PROPORTION OF MEDICAL MEN, WHOSE SERVICES WOULD NO LONGER BE REQUIRED.

The first Government with vision and faith to become a focal point for the people's good-will, and to challenge hypocrisy and exploitation, however formidable and deep-rooted, need have no misgivings. They will be violently attacked and obstructed; but, with the cards on the table and the people convinced of their sincerity, they will never hack for support. Perhaps we may yet see, in New Zealand, the first real democracy.

CAUTION!

Reform begins with the individual. There is no lack of those who want the other fellow to change *his* ways. But there is still a dearth of people determined, at whatever the cost, to subordinate their capabilities, limitations, interests, and beliefs, unreservedly, to the guidance and discipline of Omnipotent Spirit. Yet ONLY so can the NEW AGE be born.

APOLOGY.

This book makes no sort of pretension to finality. It represents merely the elementary glimmerings of life-giving truth perceptible to present spiritual measure, standard, or "time." Nothing herein is original, unless it be the manner of presentation. A Principle is involved, of universal application; and an attempt has been made, in the limited time at disposal, to co-relate the various factors hearing on health and disease, and to reduce to intelligible terms the usual vague misconceptions of what constitutes spiritual healing.

It is consoling to reflect that, through faith and discipleship, with the Spirit of Truth to teach, measure will be increased.

"For I am not ashamed of the gospel of Christ (the Spirit within); for it is the power of God (Universal Spirit of GOOD) to every one that believeth."

THE "NEW WAY."

Not many years since, during a stage of self-sufficiency of physical wisdom and wide spiritual deflection, there come into the writer's hands a book called *The Light of the Sevens*, published in 1925 by one L. E. Bassett. This book might, for all the sense it seemed, then, to him to contain, as well have been written in

Arabic. So it was dismissed, contemptuously, as the unintelligible wanderings of a disordered mind.

About a year after my change of direction from a course almost wholly physical to one less unspiritual, the author of that book was, by a spiritual apparent coincidence, encountered in person. Against the advice of friends, and not without some trepidation and misgiving, in response to an inward urge, a course of personal instruction at his hands was entered upon.

Throughout the year 1934 my new friend laboured, for hours every Sunday morning, and at many other times, to develop my grasp of new PRINCIPLE. This teaching was not in terms of (still valuable) tuition of college and university days—much of this was invalidated thereby—but in deeper spiritual cosmic PRINCIPLE; to which such tuition must be aligned and centred.

Pondering, through strenuous days, "how knoweth this man, never having learned?" there were made clear, within the relativity of spiritual cosmic PRINCIPLE, new aspects of truth.

I learned of spiritual plan, process and purpose; of the Adamic Race "World orders"; of the progressive duality of consciousness; of the Adamic "Seven Times"; of the Adamic gamut; of the positive and negative interactions; of the "Seasons" of the "Times"; of the cycles, epochs, crises, chronology, sequence, and the paradoxes of spiritual physics; of the Semitic and Japhetic parallels; of the Adamic spectra; and of much more. I learned something, also, of spiritual, mental, and physical paradoxes in vital relationship to medical science and practice.

Awakened thus to new consciousness, I "press on to the prize of the high calling," in an attempt, according to type of consciousness, to de-phase and spread the new aspects of truth; and, though many will "set at naught," others will "follow the gleam."

Passages in my book specially reflecting my friend's teachings are acknowledged by appending his initials (L.E.B.). A prediction is ventured that, in time perhaps soon to come, as my friend's teachings are more clearly grasped, the enlightened will understand, gratefully, that not all God's prophets lived yesterday.

Foreword to Fifth Edition
Health and Healing in the New Age
(1949)

"The path of the just is as the shining light, that shineth more and more unto the perfect day.

"The way of the wicked is as darkness; they know not at what they stumble."

Proverbs IV, 18 & 19.

GOD, the "Father", is infinite, divine life. This infinite life is focussed and centred in and radiates through Jesus the Christ, as the first manifestation of the infinite, unmanifest.

These propositions are advanced tentatively, not dogmatically, because, (it is submitted), recognition of them both, alone can provide either adequate incentive, or power, for man to master primitive urges, instincts and conditioned beliefs, and submit himself effectively to direction by Divine intelligence.

Life proceeds from its infinite source. All life's manifestations are vibratory; and vary according to vibratory arrangement, rate, and polarity. Since expression of the infinite in the relative is governed by spiritual science, knowledge of this science is vital. No less vital are conformity and control; otherwise man with his unlimited possibilities, and driven by potentially limitless power, is uncontrolled.

Won't we, or can't we see? Why are leaders and their flocks so inevitably and actively hostile to true science? — is it ignorance, or stupidity; impulse, or conditioning; emotion, or prejudice?

Human, mechanical, natural man, with his emotions, mind, physical body, and animal characteristics, is a product of his environment. His consciousness is limited at first to that very restricted band, low in the vibratory scale, with which his five physical senses make contact.

Human mind, manifesting through a material mechanism, cannot reason intelligently. The human mind records, and can reproduce, vibratory impressions. These, together with the product of their association, are termed "thoughts." In earliest "times," or evolutionary stages of Adamic man, mind is only very slightly, and intermittently, responsive to higher rhythms of intelligence. As man evolves, his original dim fluctuating glimmer of light, or intelligence, gradually brightens.

If spirit, God, could be said to have qualities or attributes, they might be summed as intelligence. Divine intelligence is that infinite faculty, comprising all knowledge, wisdom and understanding, which alone can discriminate between right and wrong, or tell true from false.

Intellect is materialistic. It is almost solely the sum and product of misinterpretations of distorted sense impressions recorded in human mind.

Individually or internationally, only to the degree that natural, human man subordinates intellect, instinct and emotion, to control and illumination by divine intelligence, can man become anything but a disease, or his affairs chaotic.

Mere idealism is not enough. Idealism, misaligned as to science, is destructive in proportion to deflection and motivating energy.

Nor is "religion" necessarily a guide. Intellectual misconceptions of theological science are among the world's worst curses. Religion, as commonly purveyed, is mostly the unconscious hypocrite's excuse for behaving unintelligently.

Men "turn to God"—do we? God, Spirit, expresses through principle, science, and law; knowledge of and obedience to which are the test, and most convincing evidence of sincerity. "He that hath my commandments" (knows my laws) "and keepeth" (obeys) "them, he it is that loveth me," said the Lord Jesus.

The British Commonwealth "prays" fervently, for peace and well being; and persists hitherto unrepentant, in most of the unintelligent urges and beliefs that breed poverty, war, and disease. "Not everyone that saith unto me Lord, Lord, shall enter the kingdom of heaven," cautioned Jesus the Christ, "but he that doeth the will of my Father which is in heaven."

Not all alliances are of spiritual affinity; and before this world conflict of the 20th century reaches its zenith, the British Commonwealth will be reduced to genuine repentance: real self-submission to Spirit, God—evidenced by knowledge of, and obedience to, principle, science and law.

Until this happens, chaos is like to become increasingly chaotic, confusion worse confounded.

Meanwhile, the world epoch sweeps on with ever gathering momentum towards its stupendous climax. Aggressive militarism and the Babylonic economic system, mutually dependent and destructive, are being destroyed. (The manner of their destruction, by spiritual superimposure, not many foresee.)

Ruthless, cunning sponsors of unprincipled systems—religious, educational, financial, medical, commercial, agricultural, political—fight frantically to stave off the inevitable. Suggestion and compulsion are their weapons; spiritual intelligence and power must be ours.

God's spirit and law are vindicating themselves. The Gospel of Christ is blazing forth with new light. Wholeness, individual, national, and international, are on offer—God's gift; on His terms.

The world conflict is between Divine intelligence, Christ control—and human impulse and intellect. Be of good cheer—man's deliverance from self-made miseries is part of God's purpose. The victory will be Christ's.

Ten years ago—in 1939—the fourth edition of this book appeared. Already, thousands of wonderful regenerations, by its help, attest the life-giving power of God and His Christ.

Eighteen years ago, the writer was an ordinary medical practitioner, orthodox trained, serving on the honorary surgical staff of a provincial hospital. He led a deflective existence, without the remotest suspicion that medical teaching might be defective, or that anything in this book so much as existed.

Imminence of retribution compelled a turn, away from dissipated living, towards God. A year elapsed before divine intelligence, flickering in the darkness of intellect, began to cause vague disquiet as to adequacy of medical methods and ideas. Gradually light filtered through. Every new realisation meant an inward struggle against instinctive and conditioned objection; but daily it grew clearer that something was radically and fundamentally wrong.

Within four years it was plain beyond doubt that a great percentage of teaching at the world's greatest medical schools, by the greatest "scientists," was not merely not truth—its relationship with truth was distortion, inversion, and negation. Yet youthful minds are still crammed with ever more deluding elaborations of this human, travesty of true science.

The reason is—centring of human consciousness in the physical-intellectual. The inexorable demand of this intensifying "world" epoch is elevation of the centre of consciousness and response to Christ, the spiritually-intelligent. In proportion as this is achieved will upside-down systems be revolutionised; and poverty, misery, disease, disaster, and death, give place to goodness, health, happiness, peace, security, prosperity, and life.

1. What Disease is, and How it is Brought About

"There be many that perish in this life, because they despise the Law of God that is set before them. For God hath given straight commandment to such as came, what they should do to live, even as they came, and what they should observe to avoid punishment. Nevertheless they were not obedient unto Him; but spake against Him AND IMAGINED VAIN THINGS; and deceived themselves by their wicked deeds; and said of the most High, that He is not; and knew not His ways; but His Law have they despised, and denied His covenants; in His statutes have they not been faithful, and have not performed His works. AND THEREFORE, for the empty are empty things; and for the full are the full things."

2 Esdras VII, 20-25.

GOOD HEALTH is not an entity—something to be bought or obtained. Good Health is an outward EXPRESSION of harmony with, and obedience to, the SPIRIT AND LAW OF LIFE.

Both Spirit and Law manifest polarity: they have their positive and negative aspects; so that God (Good) is positive, and evil (devil) is negative. Disease, which is ill-health, is the negative of positive, Good Health. Many people are sick because they are negative; and we are negative because we allow negative thoughts in our minds, and negative foods in our bodies. To be well, we must be or become POSITIVE.

The most important truth for man to comprehend, in fact the only consideration that really matters, is his relationship with Infinite Spirit; for everything else is dependent thereupon.

The purpose of Good Health is to enable Spirit perfectly to manifest, through perfected mental and physical vehicles; so that God's Kingdom may come, and His will be done in earth as it is in the spiritual.

MAN'S DWELLING PLACE.

We live in a marvellous house. A drug taken in at the mouth may appear on the skin of the extremities in a few minutes; a tiny quantity of poison absorbed from the intestine may throw a powerful person into convulsions; within limits, we can survive surprising extremes of heat and cold; an emotion can strike us dead, or restore us to activity; and not one atom of our make up is beyond the influence of Spirit. The Power, who designed the miracle of the human body, was not inept and likely to overlook provision for its maintenance in health. Are we to believe that God created this wonder, with its infinite complexity of reaction, and left it at the mercy of the first, or any, hostile germ that happened to cross its path? No. He conditioned that, exclusive of life's evolutionary epochs, health, whether of mind or body, might as a rule be maintained, in obedience to the laws concerned; and that if, through ignorance or perversity, we fail to obey the laws, and health in consequence is impaired, it could, usually, be regained through repentance and conversion to the Law. God's Spirit is our Life Force. "In Him we live and move and have our being." He tends to keep us in health. But if, through error or sin, health is impaired, HE is still our Life Force, still radiating well-being, and so tending powerfully, to restore us to health—when we cease thinking and doing the things that were making us ill.

SINS OF COMMISSION.

For too long we have thought like idiots, fed like fools, and acted like knaves; and then swallowed poisons or had pieces cut out of us in the hope of ridding ourselves of the consequences.

But both in the ranks of the medical profession and outside it, there is a growing realization that the phrase "Etiology obscure," is merely the refuge of the ignorant. Sir William Osler, the late world-famous physician, once said: "We put drugs, about which we know little, into our bodies, about which we know less, to cure disease, about which we know nothing at all." What an admission! Man exists out of all mental harmony with the One Source of Life; he makes his body the repository of decaying flesh mid denatured foods; he introduces into it poisons in the form of tobacco, tea, alcohol, sugar, sera, and drugs; he stuffs and gluts it with almost incredible quantities of rubbish, got up to appeal to his senses; he no longer eats to live, he lives to eat; and the temple of the Holy Ghost is befouled, and its existence endangered in order that he may continue to gratify his perverted appetites; and when the Inevitable consequences appear, the devout fold their ignorant hands and murmur, "It is the will of God," and together with the more secular, fly to the modern Medicine Man, and importune him to exorcise, with medicine or knife the mysterious devil which has crossed them!

If there existed — there does not and never will — the man who could cure by medicine or surgery, and immunise by vaccine,
HE WOULD BE THE GREATEST ENEMY OF MAN WHO EVER LIVED.

SYMPTOMS — THEIR DUAL SIGNIFICANCE.

Insufficient distinction has been drawn between symptoms and the disease process that gives rise to them. Practically our whole system of diagnosis, prevention, and treatment, has been based upon a misconception that mistakes symptoms for disease.

Symptoms are of dual significance. They are Nature's warnings of deflection from "the Law"; they are also evidence of Nature's method of cure. In either case, the more effectively we suppress them, without adequate attention to the underlying disease process and the causes that brought it about, the more effectually may we prevent Nature from achieving her beneficent purpose of protecting us from the consequences of ignorance and neglect.

The presence of disease is manifested by symptoms. These are Nature's shouted warnings; wig-wags; fog-signals; "LOOK OUT! LOOK OUT!" they warn; "you are heading for trouble!" Along comes a medicine man, misinformed as to the nature of these symptoms, and how they are caused, tears up the wig-wag, muffles the signals, silences the warnings; and so, while the danger still rushes upon him, deludes the victim into a false and frequently fatal sense of security.

COSTLY BLUNDERING.

But there is worse to follow. When, through relying upon denatured and adulterated foods, long continued over-eating, indulgence in drugs and other extraneous poisons, pandering to perverted appetite, slackness in healthy habits, constipation, and wrong mental outlook, the TOXIC TIDE IS RISING, Nature takes the situation in hand. She makes us ill—too ill to eat (if we are wise)—while she eliminates (if we will let her), through the usually adequate channels she has provided for the purpose, the poisonous accumulations that were endangering life. An outline will be given later of the part played by Fasting, in ignoring which, we deprive ourselves of Nature's most effective therapeutic expedient. Along comes the medicine man again, and insufficiently aware of the significance of these new symptoms, summons all his resources in an effort to suppress them. When he succeeds, which fortunately is not often, he has merely prevented Nature from achieving her beneficent object, and so laid a foundation for the chronic manifestations which are the despair alike of sufferer and physician.

NOT INTERESTED.

Professional men are not alone to blame. The public knows and mostly cares much less than they, what is the true explanation of their symptoms. Resentful of inconvenience, and impatient of advice or reproof, if one medical man will not summarily despatch the symptom, they run to another who will; but trying to "get well quick" is as illusory as trying to "get rich quick."

THEN AND NOW.

People sometimes wonder why Christ didn't refer more to food. But the Jews, to whom, in the great Semitic Epoch of nineteen hundred years ago, He specifically came, were people for the most part of exceedingly abstemious habit, living under Mosaic law. They had not invented the vicious practice of food processing. Bodies were sick because souls were sick. Sin was the usual cause. To the devastating effects of soul sickness, we, today, have added a calamitous Accession of wretchedness through running amok with physical Law. As the spiritual challenge of the intensifying Epoch develops, the unhappy consequences of error and Min will be magnified.

Almost all disease begins in the soul. The greater proportion of physical disharmony is but an out-picturing of discord far deeper. Hence the futility of attempting, by attacking the physical symptoms, to deal with the problems of disease.

Do not be unduly concerned with getting rid of your symptoms—SEARCH MIND AND SOUL FOR THEIR CAUSE. Better still, strive to deepen your spiritual consciousness; for full consciousness of higher relationship obliterates every disharmony.

Sick bodies could not be healed of old while souls remained sick (neither can ours); and no earthly power can heal sick souls. ONLY THE REDEMPTIVE EFFECT OF DIVINE LOVE CAN DO THAT, AND THEN ONLY THROUGH OUR REPENTANCE AND WILLING COOPERATION; AND DIVINE LOVE WITHIN IS ALWAYS STRIVING TO HEAL.

DEFECTIVE POLARIZATION.

Any system of treatment that reckons without all these considerations, is like an ecclesiastic organization that cannot translate its tenets into healing of troubles physical, economic, and international. Both resemble an electrical or engineering plant, which, having at its disposal unlimited power, through defective polarization cannot adequately express it in terms of service. Faith healing by those in whom the Spirit of the Ideal outruns the Law, and mental systems that deny the existence or relativity of matter, or contravene the Law, must be entered in the same category.

2. Disease Defined; The Cause of Disease

DISEASE, when in negative incidence, whether of body, mind, soul, or estate, whether in the individual or the mass, is mostly:

A GRADUAL DEGENERATIVE PROCESS

due to failure to comply with the requirements of wellbeing.

Of this process, ACUTE ILLNESS is commonly NATURE'S METHOD OF CURE. Disease is bodily, mental, or economic DIS-EASE.

The causes of disease may be divided into PRIMARY and SECONDARY causes.

THE PRIMARY CAUSES

There are three great fundamental requirements of good health:

1. A confident, quiet, contented, and health-conscious mind.
2. Moderation, wise choice, and correct combination of foods.
3. Healthy general habits.

These are consequent upon and expressive of right relationship with the One Source of Life.

Correspondingly, there are two great Primary Causes of Disease:

1. PSYCHOLOGICAL, due to Wrong Thinking; and resulting, besides progressive mental deterioration and possible eventual collapse, in endocrine and sympathetic dysfunction, externalizing as discordant physical vibration and physical disease.
2. PHYSICAL, due to Wrong Feeding, and Wrong Habits and Actions, resulting in:
    (a) Toxic accumulation, partly metabolic, partly absorbed from a fermenting and putrefying residue in the intestines, partly the result of pandering to perverted taste, and partly introduced as "specifics" for "treatment" of symptoms.
    (b) Vitamin and Mineral Starvation; associated with acidosis and 'infection' by bacteria—scavengers, whose activities are limited largely by the pathogenic *material* available.

All or any of these are concomitant with and indicative of an insufficiently harmonious relationship with the One Source of Life.

THE ULTIMATE CAUSE OF DISEASE, in almost every instance, is failure, by ourselves and our forbears, to obey the psychological or physical law. The reason for failure to obey the Law is insufficient response to the SPIRIT of Whom the Law is an outward expression. The reason for insufficient response is defective consciousness.

While widespread disorder is due to "spiritual-mental-physical changes manifesting in evolutionary travail, particularly at accelerated speed in this fruitional cycle," the *ultimate* root of practically all trouble is:

DEFECTIVE SPIRITUAL-COSMIC CONSCIOUSNESS, SENSITIVITY, RECEPTIVITY AND RESPONSE.

THE SECONDARY CAUSES

There are many secondary, subsidiary, or contributory causes, Toxic, Economic, "Accidental," Environmental.

HEREDITY of course plays a part. The individual is one of the mass. Similarly, the single cell is a microcosm of the parent body whence it sprang. Like the individual, it carries within itself the potentialities for evil or good, differently conditioned in different instances, of the macrocosm of which it is a unit. But few need remain in bondage, indefinitely, to hereditary influence. Innate tendencies and weaknesses, whether of body or mind, may frequently be modified and overcome. Some, at least, are residual infirmities, shirked or insincerely contended with in antecedent cosmic experience. As in the case of acquired defect, the regenerative process may be gradual; but determination, pertinacity, and faith, will often work wonders.

GERMS are frequently *associated* with the disease process. They may produce or modify symptoms. Normally their function is beneficent, protective. Some are concerned with digestion; others are scavengers, facilitating removal of waste. Germs exhibit a quality strangely reminiscent of their human hosts—they tend to assume the character of their environment. It has been demonstrated repeatedly by experiment that perfectly harmless and even beneficent germs may be metamorphosed, by altering their food, into varieties of the most deadly virulence.

> "Behind the microbe there is to be sought the cause of the microbe, and this in every case is the state of the soil which permits him to flourish"—Leonard Williams.

Disease germs are a *product* of disease, and NEVER, as the Medical Profession still blindly believes, its primary cause.

Attempts at "curing" disease, in bodies blocked with food poisons, by attacks upon the germs which may be complicating the condition, kills many germs; but kills almost as many people, and can never heal disease. People with clean systems are naturally immune; but disease germs, having appeared in the unhealthy, may disseminate disease among any whom unhealthy living has rendered susceptible. But remove the cause, eliminate the accumulated waste, and germs and symptoms alike disappear.

We must concern ourselves not with the germs, but with the wrong conditions of living that make them a menace. The best way to get rid of maggots and poisonous odours is to remove the garbage and prevent its collection — not dissipate energy in futile attempts to destroy the flies.

"ACCIDENTAL" causes are often seemingly obvious. Frequently, however, the real underlying causes are much less apparent. There is no such thing as accident in the sense usually implied; there is only cause and effect. Right understanding of cause will enable us to prevent the effect.

Most people are familiar with the painful results of dislocation of joints, and the relief that comes with reduction. But too few understand the often easily correctable disabilities resulting from lesser degrees of displacement of vertebrae, particularly the upper few.

Yet, indisputable X-ray proof notwithstanding, orthodoxy derides. But orthodox medical men were ever the last to appreciate the value of discoveries relating to health and disease. They have always resisted new truth; though, when truth has finally forced itself on them, they are not slow to arrogate to themselves full credit for its discovery.

ECONOMIC causes contribute increasingly—largely because orthodox economists, financiers, bankers and statesmen, like orthodox medical men, are profoundly and fundamentally ignorant of principle: in this case, the Spirit and Law of right economics.

Men and their systems are one; for greedy and devilish thoughts make greedy and devilish systems. The Economic system, founded on debt instead of on credit, is not merely mathematically incapable of developing our vast real wealth—it limits access to wealth already produced. Evolved of greed and treachery, in turn it encourages both. Its mate is the animal nature, and their children are poverty and war.

For spiritual man to leave control of his credit in the hands of physical man is entrusting treasure to thieves. But, having altered our thoughts, we must still know how to alter our systems; for Divine Spirit cannot express save through Law, AND IT WAS NEVER THE LAW OF GOD TO CAPITALISE THE PEOPLE'S CREDIT AND MONETISE IT AS A DEBT TO A PRIVATE MONOPOLY.

EDUCATIONAL. It is surely a grave reflection on intellect that, with an educational system costing millions a year, some very few should have to devote all their time to teaching adults the A.B.C. of how to live healthily.

Young minds are strained almost to breaking point, crammed to capacity with materialistic irrelevancies, while latent spiritual attribute and resource are not merely not educated, but aborted and atrophied.

ENVIRONMENTAL causes are associated mainly with massing in towns, and with conditions obtaining there. Not shortage of materials, not shortage of labour or space, not shortage of architectural skill, but lack of vision and lack of "money," condemn men to shabby habitations. How many buildings today are not earthquake proof — and why? What may we not achieve with resource Divinely developed! Economic pressure and stark unawareness consign men to mean tenements. Selfish enslavement to base impulse and false objectives and standards constrain them to sordid pestiferous hovels. Overcrowding, vitiated air, heat, dirt, noise, smoke, tar-dust, and fumes.

Hounded by rush, stress, and anxiety; hurrying, scurrying, hunted poor sheep! Scuttling desperately about the clanging crashing avenues of big business brooded over by sinister structures wherein are enshrined the instruments of their oppression, the Sons of God solicit permission to exist!

Walk in the street of any large town, and note the number of muck-shops; drug stores; bars; tobacconists; cake, pastry, sweet, chocolate, ice cream and coloured drink vendors; all scrounging existence by trading on self-indulgence. A vast mountain of disease-causing refuse is greedily gobbled each day by vapid sensualists in search of an illusive sensation.

Primordial instinct is insistent. The ape must stuff his belly with something. The more factitious the lure, the more it seems to entice. Milk bars are the latest craze.

Picture shows supply mental pabulum, with an intellectual standard of the fourth form, and the morals of Hollywood and the Bowery.

For music: crooners and bad jazz, with cacophonous squeals, and the tom-tom thump thump of jungle fear, cruelty, lust.

Papers and periodicals, shop windows, and sky signs, neon lights and loud speakers, shriek and blare forth their lying advertisements.

We are plundered on all sides; but few see through the clumsy deceptions, or are interested enough to try. The sick cannot be induced to live healthily; but the mere mention of Boolswool's Tonic, or Kidomuk, is sufficient to separate them and their fool's pence.

The while huge sums are squandered in so-called research! Small wonder our world was dubbed, by a satirical Frenchman, the lunatic asylum of an insane universe!

Betrayed? Yes! Deluded, seduced, and corrupted; threatened, not merely with disaster, but with final extinction—by human physical wisdom.

"And thine ears shall hear behind thee a voice saying, This is the way, walk ye in it."

Isaiah, XXX, 21.

VITAMIN AND MINERAL DEFICIENCY, and TOXIC ACCUMULATION, brought about by all the above-mentioned, are the GREAT PHYSICAL, SECONDARY, CAUSE OF DISEASE.

MINERAL DEFICIENCY.

Physical life is an electro-chemical process. Not merely is the body built largely of minerals, and not merely are the blood, digestive and tissue fluids solutions of them—minerals are the body's cleansing materials for keeping it clear of waste. Despoiled of supplies, the body deteriorates.

There are seventeen minerals, such as calcium, sodium, potassium, iron, magnesium, iodine, etc., used by Nature in the construction of living tissue. They occur in our bodies in large or appreciable quantities; other trace-elements exist. They are constantly being excreted. Practically the only source of replacement is food. It is a striking reflection upon intelligence that, with good health and immunity absolutely dependent upon an adequate supply, we should go to almost every length of ingenuity to deprive ourselves of as many as we do.

Methods in vogue that partially or completely demineralise are: manufacturing, refining, processing, beautifying, peeling, freezing, canning and bottling.

Their object is mostly gain. Ignorance, stupidity, stubbornness, greed, are the stumbling blocks.

Demineralisation is coupled with unbalanced feeding—acid accumulation leeching valuable stocks, and vitamin shortage preventing absorption. Bad cooking, capricious appetite, restricted choice, parental indulgence, and mulish self-will, diminish reserves.

Foods grown in acid, deficient soil, and forced for quick sale with unnatural manures, yield scanty amounts. Inorganic minerals are no adequate substitute, in men or in soil; to ensure assimilation, minerals must be vitalised by passage through plants, or potentised by trituration.

VITAMINS are the life-element in food. They resemble faith in that very little of either is required; but without them the aliment, however liberal, cannot sustain. Many of them are modified or destroyed by heat or chemicals. Many, sometimes all, are removed by ignorant manufacturers greedy for gain. Short of its vitamins, the body gradually deteriorates; starved of most, it rapidly decays; deprived of them all, it cannot survive.

Refined foods are dead; and dead foods cannot support healthy life. Vitamin deficiency is accompanied by stunted growth, bacterial infection, toxic absorption, deformities, and ulceration; it predisposes to character distortion, mental and moral deterioration, and national and international degradation.

Examples of disease wholly or in part caused by Vitamin and Mineral Deficiency are:

Infantile Paralysis (Poliomyelitis), Tuberculosis, Rickets, Scurvy, Eczema, Anaemia, Glaucoma, Cataract, Blindness, Deafness, Goitre, Rheumatism, Neuritis, some Kidney Stones, and Cancer.

There is one certain protection against the destructive effects of devitalised foods: NEVER USE ANY.

AVOID, LIKE THE PLAGUES THEY GIVE RISE TO, WHITE FLOUR, POLISHED RICE, WHITE SUGAR, CORNFLOUR, AND ANYTHING AND EVERYTHING MADE FROM SUCH THINGS.

TOXIC ACCUMULATION.

Normally, when food is completely metabolised, the results are: growth, tissue repair, heat, energy, and waste.

This waste matter is poisonous; and comprehensive provision has been made for extrusion. A most important duty of Skin, Lungs, Liver, Kidneys, and Bowel, is ridding the body of waste. Poisons not oxidised in the tissues are carried by blood and lymph to the Eliminating Organs, strained out by them, and expelled.

Ordinarily the Eliminating System is more than capable of coping completely with waste; but if waste be introduced, or produced, of a kind or in quantity such as the body is not designed to deal with, accumulation occurs. Fermentation products from excess undigested sugar and starch, and deadly putrefactive alkaloids from rotting flesh foods, are the worst of the physical cancer-producers.

The amount and variety of noxious substances amassed in people's bodies is sometimes fantastic. The harm done ranges from mild discomfort and vague pains, to decrepitude, circulatory or nervous breakdown, vicious or criminal impulse, confusion, insanity, and death.

People, as a rule, are fairly particular about outward cleanliness; but within, the temple of God's Spirit is a dunghill : a foul and steaming cesspool of indescribable beastliness.

To avert retribution, these feculent sumps are ravaged with surgical violence, riven with drug and germ poisons, and rent with shattering thought forces.

"If any man defile the temple of God, him shall God destroy."

1 Corinthians III, 17.

"FIFTEEN POINTS" OF POLLUTION.

Prominent among the everyday causes of Toxic Accumulation are:

1. *Mental tension*, such as fear, jealousy, bitterness, hate, resentment, self-pity. In addition to the terrific battery of physical poisons, the body is often flooded, in many continuously, with its own internal secretions. Always toxic in excess, they become particularly so under the influence of dread, hate, rage, or other unrestrained emotion or wrong thought. So poisonous may be emotion that the breath of an angry man, condensed and injected, has killed a rabbit in convulsions.

2. *Overeating*, specially of cooked meat, and refined, denatured, adulterated rubbish masquerading as food.

3. *Muck-eating*, swallowing death-dealing refuse in the form of cakes and pastries made from white flour and sugar, sweets, chocolates, ice-creams, milkshakes, and coloured drinks.
4. *Self-poisoning*, with alcohol, tobacco, and drugs.
5. *Doping*, or administering poisons in the form of vaccines, sera, and "medicines," to "cure" the symptoms of Toxaemia.
6. *Adulteration*, the presence in almost everything eaten of a Machiavellian assortment of venom.
7. *Indolence* and laziness; with breathing and activity insufficient for complete oxygenation.
8. *Constipation*, because lazy habits, overloading, and not enough roughage, reinforced by mental tension and drugs, interfere with right function.
9. *Auto-intoxication*, by absorption from the intestines of the reeking emanations from fermentation, decomposition, and putrefaction.
10. *Mechanical*, where spinal subluxations cause defective innervation.
11. *Bacterial activity*, because disease germs develop in dirt; and, becoming virulent in a toxic environment, themselves evolve matter of high toxicity.
12. *Trade poisoning*, where workers in anilin, paraffin, lead, munitions, etc., become cancerous, blinded, or paralysed.
13. *Ergotism*, through using meat, milk, butter, and cheese, from cows feeding on ergotised pastures; and, in New Zealand, pastures are riddled with ergot from end to end of the land. This also explains much mysterious stock disease. (A. Kent.)

14. *Aluminium poisoning*, an insidious trap for the unwary. Minute portions of aluminium utensils, used in the preparation of foods, are absorbed as hydroxide; and, though apparently innocuous, are deadly in course of time.

15. *Chronic Acid Poisoning: Acidosis*, the International Endemic. Meats, starches, sugars, and animal fats are the great acid-producers. That is to say, assimilated and metabolised, the residual waste is acid in character — carbonic acid, uric acid, and a variety of complex organic acids. These are mostly sparingly soluble, and consequently difficult of elimination. Combination with alkaline minerals increases solubility and eliminability.

THE CALCIUM THIEVES.

For successful elimination of acid residue from sugar and starch metabolism, CALCIUM is required. If the supply is inadequate, or if this waste is produced in excess, the acids accumulate. To combat this, the body calls up its calcium reserves from teeth and bones, which, gradually or rapidly, become de-calcified, crumble, and rot.

This is one very important reason why New Zealanders, who consume inordinate amounts of meat, sugar, and starch, have the worst teeth and brittlest bones in the world; and, incidentally, one of the highest cancer death-rates. Concomitant upset of calcium-phosphorus ratio results in arteriosclerosis, rheumatism, gout, and a host of degenerative manifestations.

Filching from cereals and other foods the protective alkaline minerals, and throwing them to the pigs, while we attempt the impossible task of living healthily on the acid-forming starch left behind, *may, and does, make good pigs; but makes very bad human beings!*

Why be uncharitable to the defenceless, small germs?

3. Orthodox Medical Methods Cause Disease

"And a certain woman . . . had suffered many things of many physicians, and had spent all that she had, and was nothing bettered, but rather grew worse."

Mark V, 26.

WHAT follows is an impersonal survey. Neither individuals; nor associations of individuals are arraigned. Methods, not men, are to blame. A vital principle is involved. The charge must be faced that misaligned medical methods, far from solving the disease problem, have become, in fact, the second in importance of its two principal causes.

There are two GREAT REASONS for the existence and persistence of Chronic Disease:

1. *Continuing to think, eat, or do the things that make people ill.*
2. *Suppressing Nature's curative efforts.*

Those who are ill and wish to get well can do so, most of them, subject to one absolute condition:

That they think, eat, and act aright; and co-operate loyally with Nature's efforts to heal.

There are five hundred thousand sick people in New Zealand; and five hundred thousand more are not as well as they should be. Of the remainder, hardly a handful even approaches the ideal. The thoughtful may well ask—why don't the doctors cure them? And the answer is, not only do orthodox methods not CURE disease, but in too many instances they aggravate or actually cause disease and prevent recovery.

THINK! (If "education" has not completely incapacitated.) How can orthodox medical men "cure" disease? They do not even know what disease is, nor how it is caused; still less have they understood the Natural or Spiritual resources for prevention or treatment.

That there is a disease problem, no one need argue. The urgent demand for rapidly expanding hospital and asylum accommodation, and the proposed fantastic expenditure of debt money, sufficiently attest the fact. But if problems are to be solved, they must be considered in principle; otherwise, attempts at solution, however well-intentioned, must fall far short.

The world is in an epoch of cosmic accelerating intensity that DEMANDS a new spiritual alignment; with increasing sensitivity, receptivity, and response.

"IN WHOM THE GOD OF THIS WORLD . . ."

No minds are more holden, today, than those still blinded, despite proven futility, by belief in the adequacy of human physical wisdom. In deflection from principle, orthodox methods have failed catastrophically; and this deflection is symptomatic and characteristic of defective spiritual-cosmic consciousness. Both physically and spiritually, man is evolving; but even in this transitional stage of a world order now rapidly drawing to a close, humanity Adamic response is still far too limited to the physical-intellectual. The emerging new order DEMANDS a higher response.

ORTHODOX METHODS NEVER "CURE" DISEASE.

Orthodox methods have failed, principally because, insufficiently comprehending Spirit as the one constituent of Life and all matter, we have regarded as physical, problems always ultimately spiritual. Consequently, we have looked without, for cause and cure of troubles arising within.

Looking without, for the cause of disease, there were discovered, not merely associated with the disease process, but capable sometimes even of propagation, minute living organisms or "disease-germs." It was erroneously, though quite naturally, concluded that these were the cause.

Enlightened reflection, however, discloses that "disease-germs" are merely one factor—usually an effect—and NEVER the primary cause. *The primary cause of almost all disease is failure to fulfil the requirements of well-being.*

Thus the "healing" system, like the financial system founded on debt instead of on credit, begins upside down. Both systems are based on a false premise, upon which vast inverted pyramids have been built. The time has come to kick out the bottom brick, and rebuild.

SYMPTOMS AND DIAGNOSIS.

"Symptoms are of dual significance. They are Nature's warnings of deflection from 'the Law'; they are also evidence of Nature's method of cure. In either case, the more effectively we suppress them, without adequate attention to the underlying disease process and the causes that brought it about, the more effectually may we prevent Nature from achieving her beneficent purpose of protecting us from the consequences of ignorance and neglect."

Not understanding, we have feared disease and sought to get rid of it by doping, cutting, and burning its symptoms. The uncured imagine, and are encouraged to believe that they are merely among the unfortunate whose difficulties have not yet been fathomed by medical "science." They certainly are, inasmuch as practically every sick individual has to be included in the same category.

Orthodox "diagnosis" means little more than giving symptoms a name; very often, as experience has demonstrated, a wrong one. It has been proved that the most skilful diagnostician, with all the resources of a modern hospital at his disposal, is correct in only forty-eight per cent of cases in even naming the symptoms; and naming the symptoms does nothing to reveal the true cause.

Unlike those who approach problems in principle, orthodoxy cannot institute "treatment" without "diagnosis"; and much wrong treatment is done to obviate the otherwise monotonous regularity of the too damaging admission—"nothing can be done." "Do zummat," is the motto of the old school.

For such reasons, all manner of disastrous "treatment," including tens of thousands of expensive, painful, and mutilating operations, is undertaken, often on no better pretext than a bad guess.

"Observation" and "investigation" are ingenious (and usually exorbitantly expensive) resources, whose chief usefulness lies in concealing from the sufferer his physician's ignorance of what ails him. Fear and disease-consciousness, "examination" engendered, are among the worst causes of disease. Lacking the principle, the would-be helper is in no better case than his patient; and when the blind lead the blind, both fall into the ditch.

There is no "cure" for disease. Recovery comes through faith and obedience. The struggle for self-mastery may be deferred; but cannot be evaded. One of our crimes has been the proffering of illusory palliatives.

True diagnosis consists in discovering the barriers, both psychological and physical, preventing the divine Life Force within from manifesting perfection. Naming the symptoms is seldom important. Effective treatment consists in helping the afflicted to remove all barriers; and in encouraging a higher consciousness and response. *There is a whole world of difference between mechanical treatment of symptoms in the well-to-do; and a protracted and exacting wrestle with sick, weak, ignorant, stubborn, fearful, penurious souls.*

THE INVARIABLE MISTAKE.

The first great departure from principle is made when doctors, insufficiently responsive to divine Spirit and Law, look IN SICK BODIES FOR CAUSES. They never discover them; for the primary cause is never in the body, that's where effects appear. The cause will be found in the mind or the manner of living. Error at the very outset has limited us to battling with effects, and the further we have gone the more have we retrogressed.

FAMILIAR SUPPRESSIVE MEASURES.

Repeatedly and consistently to thwart Nature's curative efforts is bad enough when one knows no better; to continue to do so, enlightened, is criminal idiocy; to employ means to that end demonstrably destructive and disease-producing in themselves, is surely to plumb the last depths of human futility.

Familiar orthodox expedients for suppressing the symptoms of disease are Drugs; Vaccines and Sera; Surgical Operations; Radium and X-Rays. Almost invariably these are inherently deadly. Not merely may they bring low the most powerful; their employment conceals the path along which alone deliverance lies.

Almost all drugs are poisonous. Many are venomous. Few are even temporarily admissible. None would be required if natural requirements were complied with. Were we not taught not to "think," the stupidity of swallowing or injecting noxious substances with a view to ridding ourselves of the consequence of wrong thinking and living, would hardly need emphasis.

Agranulocytosis (in plain language, low white blood cell count), is a fatal disorder whose origin had long been a mystery. It is now known to be caused by Pyramidon, a drug taken and widely prescribed by "specialists," for relieving symptoms derived from elementary errors in the manner of living. [Pyramidon is an analgesic now banned in many countries, S.A.H.B.]

Sir William Wilcox, the eminent English toxicologist, in the *British Medical Journal* in the 1930s, disclosed that this disastrous disease is caused also by the salicylates (e.g. aspirin) — drugs universally taken and prescribed by medical men the world over, for the suppression of symptoms they call "rheumatism." But such symptoms are no more than commonplace consequences of wrong feeding and general habits — not infrequently, of unhappiness merely.

Agranulocytosis may also be caused by the barbiturates (Luminal [phenobarbitone], the great brain paralyser, was the best known), prescribed literally in tons for suppressing nervous symptoms arising from toxic conditions of body and mind. [Although barbiturates are largely out of favour for this use in the 21st century, toxic psychiatric medications such as the SSRIs are now widely prescribed, S.A.H.B.]

Also, says Sir William, by "Avertin," used as a basal anaesthetic in surgical operations for cutting out symptoms amenable often to simple natural methods.

ALSO BY ASPIRIN! Who dare compute the number of tons of this potent destroyer swallowed annually to relieve the symptoms of stupid living?

One English firm spent £340,000, in one year, in advertisement alone, on one particular futile disease-producer.

(Equivalent to £17,000,000 in 2022.)

And the *British Medical Journal* continues to draw large sums from advertising, to medical men, the poisons its own columns condemn! [Now the columns support the poisons!, S.A.H.B.]

What Sir William Wilcox has yet to discover is, as every Naturopath knows, that agranulocytosis is only one of the killing effects of the above named poisons. Presently it will dawn on him, to his horror and dismay, that deafness, eczema, asthma, blindness, paralysis, criminal degeneracy, delusions, cancer, and insanity, together with numerous other appalling adversities, quite frequently eventuate from a variety of drugs so comprehensive as to include almost the whole range. These are reckoned already by tens of thousands; and are continually increasing in numbers, futility, and toxicity.

Not long ago, while eulogies appeared of "God's G. men," as a paper was pleased to term us medical men, a paragraph recorded some hundreds of deaths caused by the latest drug advocated to "cure" "blood-poisoning."

Inept in their ignorance, though anxious enough to aid, those who prescribe these compounds know practically nothing of their composition, and less of their action. immediate or remote. Desperate in their helplessness, and beguiled by specious and cunningly worded advertisement, they clutch at the subtle deceptions as a drowning man at a straw; they impose upon public confidence by prescribing on the say-so of salesmen carefully trained to take advantage of ignorance and credulity.

Doctors thus become the agents for destroyers more frightful than phosgene.

VACCINES AND SERA.

Even if objective evidence, in reaction, sickness and death, were lacking (which it is not), that vaccines and sera can cause disease, no very profound depth of intelligence is needed to envisage the ingenuousness of injecting the filthy products of disease into a healthy person to keep him well. At best, such conduct is a cynical reflection on Divine Spirit and Law.

Again in the *British Medical Journal* one medical man recorded 16 cases, in his own practice alone, of paralysis following preventive (!) injection of "diphtheria antitoxin," in people who had never suffered from the "disease." The query must be urged — how many cases of paralysis, then, follow its "therapeutic" use in all the hospitals of the "civilised" world? And since paralysis is but one of its possible sequelae, the curious may speculate as to the real extent of the harm.

The cream of the joke is, of course, there's no such disease! "Diphtheria" is the name of a symptom. Acute sore throats are evidence of Nature's healing reaction — certainly preventible by healthy living; and quickly responding to fasting.

If germs are so terrible, why do these acute so-called "infective" disorders yield so dramatically to fasting and simple elimination? If the germ were the relevant factor, fasting would surely be fatal. Appreciation of this point will soon close our "fever-traps."

If germs were the fearful menace the apostles of orthodoxy allege, vaccines and sera might be a logical, if flimsy defence. But, as minds not inaccessible to truth will perceive. the healthy do not succumb. Disease being established, disease germs may appear. Yet in America and England, the medical associations are striving for absolute autocracy; one object being compulsory "immunisation" against "diphtheria" and other "diseases." As if immunisation were possible by inoculation with disease, against the disciplinary consequences of indulgent living!

A number of children were killed in Australia, quite recently, by vaccines; and a larger number in Chicago. These regrettable incidents were hushed up by interested parties; and the vaccines responsible exonerated. [This is in reference to events in the 1930s but the harm of vaccines continues today, S.A.H.B.]

Epidemics of cholera in destitute countries are attributed by orthodoxy to germs. (Many varieties are described; but better counting will equate the varieties with the number of sufferers.) And so the germs are attacked. But the educational, economic, and religious systems, responsible for the filthy living conditions and inadequate diet that cause the disease, are allowed to remain unchallenged.

Great capital has been made, by protagonists of the germ theory, out of the apparent reduction of typhoid incidence in the Great War. True, by suppressive methods, the form of disease may be changed; but that does not arrest the disease process — of which acute illness is curative. Statistics can be made to prove anything; but any reduction was due to improved hygiene, not to anti-typhoid inoculation, which sickened and killed enough. Moreover, "new diseases," labelled "paratyphoid A and B," "trench fever," "P.U.O.," pyrexia (of unknown origin!) etc., were handy designations concealing the fact that the old familiar consequences of unhealthy living had merely altered their name.

Pasteur was the first to misinterpret, commercialise, and exploit, at the expense of ignorant sufferers, the discoveries of wiser and better men—Antoine Béchamp, for example. Today, Pasteur is the great false god of disease.

Pasteur was the fore-runner of modern bug-factories, with millions invested, producing ludicrous and unpredictable dirt differing more in name than in kind from the preposterous concoctions of an age scarce gone. Shiploads are sent out. A vast business of trafficking in human misery has been built up. Behind the medical men and their hospitals is a colossal organization, profit-inspired, for making and marketing drugs, vaccines, surgical supplies, and dead foods. And only too often doctors are the unpaid salesmen!

Who controls all this capital? Who controls any capital? Who really controls banking and vested interests? Those who control money and credit control most else. Is it too fantastic to suggest that the people are victims of a grand-scale conspiracy, among whose dupes are the medical men?

SURGICAL OPERATIONS.

There is still a legitimate, though narrow and rapidly contracting, field for surgery. At best, it is symptom-swatting, concerned exclusively with effects. There can hardly be a diseased organ in an otherwise healthy body; and permanent good has seldom resulted from excising the unhealthiest portions, and leaving the rest diseased.

When the cause of ill-health is dietetic, "exploratory" operating is turpitude; when psychological, "having a gink" is little better than homicide. Says the surgeon, "there's something wrong somewhere; let's have a look-see"; or, "something's amiss, let's cut it out."

But blundering interference with structure and function, though faultlessly intentioned, must reap a sorry reward. Masking of symptoms deludes. It prevents recognition of error; and, too frequently, delays or aborts Nature's curative purpose.

The vast majority of symptoms are either psychological or dietetic in origin; and readily respond when the cause is corrected. By subjecting them indiscriminately, often by sadly incompetent performers, to painful and useless violence, trivial complaints are converted into serious and intractable disorder. And surgery is by no means the only field of activity where ignorance, ineptitude, and calamitous failure are rewarded with thanks, high honour, and rich fees.

Operations, unfortunately, are among the most lucrative items of the orthodox stock-in-trade. They must be sold, otherwise it is improbable that people will buy. The people, rightly, fear operations. But they can be made to fear sickness more, and the fear-urge is widely employed.

The writer was orthodox trained and served on the honorary surgical staff of a provincial hospital. Following spiritual realignment (of exigency, because of delinquency) new understanding dawned. Gradually he was made aware that something was radically and fundamentally amiss with what he had been taught, practised for fourteen years, and till then never doubted. Hardly a thought in this article but was outside his consciousness four years ago.

Developing experience of Nature's way has convinced that at least eighty per cent of operations could forthwith he dispensed with. Dr Charles Mayo, and other authorities, have put the figure at ninety per cent.

Eighty-five per cent of appendices removed have nothing the matter with them. The remainder do best left alone. Appendicitis, peritonitis, osteomyelitis, hernia, displacements, fibroids, cancer, antrum, sinus and mastoid disease, unhealthy tonsils, pyorrhoea, gall-stones, and inflammation of the gall-bladder, goitre, kidney-stones, abscesses, enlarged prostates and tumours are among the conditions usually regarded as surgical which have been shown to yield, sometimes very easily, to the simplest of natural methods.

There are innumerable instances of people having been operated upon two, three, five, ten, twenty, and even more times. But how many regain or maintain good health thereby?

It's the people's affair. If they like paying through the nose to be slaughtered in battalions — that's their privilege, of course; but if it is health they are seeking, it is dangerous to look for it at the hands of those who trade mainly in disease.

THE TONSIL AND APPENDIX RACKET.

Tens of thousands of appendices, and hundreds of thousands of tonsils are removed annually without colour of real excuse.

The cause of unhealthy tonsils is unhealthy living — faulty feeding and general habits. Tonsils and adenoids are accessory eliminating channels. Do not seal them up; correct the unhealthy living and, in course of time, the diseased condition will recover.

Yet we find school health (!) officers, while completely ignoring the causes, actually threatening to exclude children from school unless they are subjected to this useless AND DANGEROUS mutilation.

APPENDICITIS is caused by constipation, and fermentation and putrefaction of excess starch and, or, meat.

APPENDICITIS NEVER OCCURS IN PEOPLE OR NATIONS WHO EAT WISELY. Conservatively treated, like most other Acute Illnesses or Healing Crises, with fasting (absolute in acute attacks); rest; cold packs; and, in acute attacks, not even laxatives or enemata—there is practically no death-rate.

When the surgical treatment of appendicitis has ceased, the death-rate from this condition will cease also. It is the operation that kills—not the disorder.

THE CANCER INDUSTRY: RADIUM, X-RAYS, AND CANCER RESEARCH.

In no branch of their sorrows are the people being more cruelly and treacherously deceived and imposed upon than where this horrible scourge is concerned. It is almost beyond belief that men so well-intentioned as medical-men can be so blind; but "there are none so blind as they that will not see."

The people are urged to co-operate in exposing the false claims made for orthodox methods of treating this evil. We are continually reassured that early treatment by orthodox methods offers bright hope of cure; and that the proportion of cures is steadily growing.

SUCH STATEMENTS ARE UTTERLY MISLEADING.
THE DEATH-RATE FROM CANCER IS LEAPING AND BOUNDING UP!

Actually, apart from certain small skin sores which are not really cancers, the number of recoveries through orthodox methods is so small as to be almost non-existent. That many cases are *caused* by these methods, and many many more made much worse—and that at hideous cost in money and pain—is established fact.

THE MORTALITY PER LIVING MILLION FROM CANCER IN ENGLAND AND WALES INCREASED FROM 274 IN THE YEAR 1850 TO 1,563 IN THE YEAR 1934; AND IS STILL SWEEPING UPWARD.

People now suffering from cancer were, ten, twenty, and thirty years ago, *exactly as the younger people are today*! The disease process that ends as a cancerous growth, or some other of the killing disorders, gives warning throughout its course by symptoms. "Symptoms are Nature's warnings!"

The tragedy of the orthodox viewpoint is that, regarding the various symptoms as different diseases prevents early recognition and arrest of the disease process that gives rise to them. If the cause of cancer be allowed in every case to continue until the growth appears, the degenerative process will always be permitted to proceed beyond the point at which it is most easily dealt with.

If anything more than the constantly and steeply soaring mortality rate were required to convince of the lamentable futility of the orthodox approach to the "cancer problem," it would be found in the reflection that, without exception, their entire armamentarium is concentrated upon trying to "cure" the growth. *But cancer is not a local "disease."* The growth is a local manifestation of constitutional disorder; and, like most other evidences of the disease process, can be effectually dealt with only when the cause is corrected.

Also, as with most other symptoms, when the cause is corrected, the effect exhibits an often astonishing tendency to disappear.

THREE FACTORS MAKE CANCER FATAL:

1. Continuation of the cause.
2. Orthodox efforts to cure.
3. Fear, and mistaken belief in incurability.

"Cancer" is but one result of failure to live healthily: *psychological turmoil, wrong thinking, vitamin and mineral deficiency, and toxic accumulation, are the causes. Faith and obedience to law are the chief remedy. With this, as with almost all other disharmony, recovery must come from within.*

Everyone knows that both radium and X-rays are capable of causing cancer. By what inversion of reasoning, then, have agents known to be causative come to be looked on as curative?

Hundreds of thousands of animals are tortured to death every year, repeatedly with fiendish and inconceivable cruelty, while men search in their pitiful pain-racked bodies for a cause that lies in the human soul! "Cancer research" has become a lucrative industry and is one of the darkest of all blots on a tarnished escutcheon.

HOSPITAL FOLLY.

Capital expenditure bordering on a million pounds, involving increased annual charges of probably over a hundred and twenty thousand pounds, is contemplated in Wellington alone for extending the local "disease-factory." Yet with better methods of prevention and treatment immediately available, existing accommodation could be reduced, now, by one half, and still further curtailed very soon. Truly, "whom the gods would destroy, they first make mad," and they don't have to work overtime.

MENTAL DISEASE.

"Man is spirit, mind, body; not separate entities but different phases of one constituent—Spirit." Therefore, logically, little understood as both of them are, mental and physical disease are due to exactly the same causes; and respond to similar treatment.

The influence of fear, of negative thought generally, of faulty compensation to major or minor psychological stress, of mental healing crises, of toxaemia, is insignificant to orthodoxy. As much in the dark as with physical disease, and unable to cut out diseased minds, we attach, as to sick bodies, neat but misleading labels. We fill the poor creatures with enough brain and soul paralysing drugs to sink the most powerful, herd them in droves, and leave it at that.

By such means the simplest of psychological mal-adjustments is often steadily, sometimes rapidly, intensified into chaotic breakdown.

Acute illness as a healing reaction is not confined to the body. It is potentially curative likewise—as well as premonitory—in mind, soul, and material circumstance. Mental disease provides no exception to the axiom that, whatever symptoms may be, the causes will almost invariably be found under one or other or both of our two primary headings—Psychological or Physical.

Blind, wilful ignorance of this principle results in diabolical mishandling of mental disorder. Thousands are incarcerated in asylums, like thugs in a dungeon, who should never have gone there. Thousands whose often quite transitory symptoms were reactions against bodily toxins, drugs, or unhappiness, many of whom, even now, could be redeemed by love and wise help, are allowed to rot, driven at last insane by the appalling conditions in which they are forced to exist.

Almost utterly ignorant of causes and significance, orthodoxy fears mental, like physical, healing crises; and the wretched creatures God is trying to heal are rushed off to the mad-house, the very haunts of devils and horror. They are fed on a diet that would destroy the most powerful, deprived of occupation, kept in a grievous condition of physical toxaemia, soaked and saturated with horrible drugs, looked upon as insane, deprived of their civil rights, and left to a frightful fate.

If ever a monstrous injustice cried to high heaven for redress, this hideous wickedness must be stopped. We are our brother's keeper! The sum of avoidable suffering is so dreadful, that if there be one iota of pity, one spark of compassion, one vestige of righteous indignation, the revealing and redeeming Light of Divine Love and Truth must be carried into these hells upon earth.

Broken-hearted appeals and cries of despair still fall on deaf ears; and in no domain of fearful affliction is orthodox authority more direly abused to retain its sinister grip and resist reform.

"IS IT NOTHING TO YOU, ALL YE THAT PASS BY?"

THE LAST STRAW.

Appalling as all this is, there is yet worse to come. Ignorant of the miraculous possibilities of positively impressing the subconscious, orthodoxy has little conception of the tragedies wrought by negative suggestion.

Generally of strong and often powerful personality, doctors' reactions are minutely observed by the anxious, suggestible sick. A word, a look, a silence, a gesture, a thought, a belief unexpressed may suffice. The patient will know. His mind will respond. The impression received may deliver him from doom or seal his fate.

Love and confidence are the very essence of the divine healing power; fear is the great destroyer. Finalising judgment, very often in error, from the restricted resources of physical-intellectual limit, medical men are continually betrayed into diagnosis, prognosis, and treatment destructive beyond compute, when an understanding word of reassurance or admonition would work miracles.

A fitting epitaph on the tombstone of orthodoxy will read, before long: *"Nothing can be done for you."*

MISALIGNED SYSTEMS.

Modern medicine is the most lunatic system ever devised by man to his own undoing, except the financial, of which it is part.

Medical methods don't cure. Their subserviency encourages indolence of body and mind. The whole tendency of orthodox medicine is to create and perpetuate sickness, and make it attractive to those lacking the moral qualities to live healthily.

We labour under paradoxical systems — "a healing system" which only too often causes disease and prevents recovery; a financial system that limits production, development of resource, and access to goods and services available; an "educational" system, that retards the higher unfoldment; and an ecclesiastical system that has become one of the great barriers to truth.

The debt system of finance causes poverty and insecurity; breeds crime and disease; foments international bitterness; and makes war inevitable.

The greatest advance towards abolishing poverty and disease would be to change all these systems. But before we can alter them, we shall have to alter ourselves; for, like physical appearances in general, our systems reflect the consciousness of those they are intended to serve. Defective spiritual-cosmic consciousness is the ultimate root of practically all our troubles.

ORTHODOX OPPOSITION.

It is useless looking to orthodoxy for reform. Orthodoxy always bitterly and relentlessly opposes reform. In every case, the favourite weapons are:

1. A conspiracy of silence concerning the truth.
2. Ridicule and disparagement.
3. Personal attacks on witnesses of truth.
4. Hostile and misleading propaganda.
5. Others more militant as the challenge develops.

The channels of publicity are mostly in the hands of the enemy. No effort is spared to throw dust in our eyes — the ignorant are easily exploited; the instructed, less readily.

We ourselves are to blame. Give the average man a crust and a corner of blanket, and he's satisfied. "It is not because tyrants oppress them that the people are slaves," said a sage, "it is because they are so abject that the powerful and unprincipled will inevitably exploit them."

Both in economics and health, in the individual and the mass, recovery must come from within. Responsive persons everywhere must rally to the imperious summons. We must learn, as the only genuinely democratic alternative to materialistic dictatorship of one kind or another, individually and collectively to govern ourselves. This we can do successfully only as we turn, in obedience to His Law, to the one Infinite Source of all wisdom, knowledge, understanding, life, health, prosperity, security, and love, immanent as well as transcendent.

4. The Problem of Treatment — General Considerations

"When Jesus heard it, he saith unto them, They that are whole have no need of the physician, but they that are sick: I came not to call the righteous, but sinners to repentance."

Mark II, 17.

I. THE DAWN OF A BETTER DAY

"And great multitudes followed Him, and He healed them ALL."

Matthew XIX, 2.

IF our interpretation of the gospel is not healing troubles of body, mind, soul, and estate, in the individual and in the mass, then our interpretation is in urgent need of revision, for THERE'S NOTHING WRONG WITH THE GOSPEL.

A vital part of the gospel of Christ is the Power around and within, able and anxious to take over, as soon as we will and to the degree of our response, control and direction of every detail of our affairs, whether of body, mind, soul, or estate, whether in the individual or the mass — to heal and sustain, to provide and protect, to counsel and inspire, to unfold our destiny and endue us with power to follow it out.

There is only One Universal Source of matter, energy, Life and GOOD — Omnipresent, Omniscient, Omnipotent, Divine, Living, Loving LIFE SPIRIT.

There is no such thing as matter apart from Spirit, of which matter is a manifestation. Matter is Spirit in relativity.

Man is being made in the image and likeness of God — perfect, whole, glorious. Misapprehension of this radiant truth, through material consciousness insufficiently developed, prevents Divine perfection from manifesting.

RELIEF, OR REFORM.

"Wilt thou be made whole," smilingly enquired the Master. Do we sincerely desire, that is, individually and collectively, not merely to have uncomfortable symptoms removed, but inwardly and outwardly to co-operate in being made *whole*? Most are perfectly willing, and anxious, to have their sufferings abated, if someone will do it for them; but voluntary submission to the change of mental outlook and physical discipline essential to real healing seems too high a price.

By far the greater proportion of ill-health is Psychological in origin, and cannot be cured by physical means. Even dietetic disorder is rooted in ignorance, stupidity, stubbornness, and greed.

There is no such thing as "cure." Disease, is mostly a degenerative process, the consequence, in ourselves or our forebears, of disobedience to spiritual-cosmic Law; healing is a regenerative process, the outcome of repentance and obedience to Law; and obedience is a fruit of harmony with the Spirit of the Law, without which, incentive, due to the weakness of the flesh, eventually proves inadequate.

Motive needs scrutiny. So many desire release from their symptoms in order to be free to indulge, unhampered, the things that are causing them. They want relief not reform. Others seek "treatment" and sympathy; not healing, at any cost. Disease is their hobby; and themselves their sole interest.

Removal or masking of symptoms does little to cure disease; though it is easier, far, and greatly more lucrative, to peddle expensive expedients than to wrestle pertinaciously with individual and mass ignorance, weakness, or viciousness.

Moreover, whatever symptoms may be, the primary cause will almost always be found under one or other, or both, of our two primary headings — Psychological or Physical; *and symptoms exhibit, often, a remarkable tendency to disappear of themselves when the cause is corrected.*

A PURPOSE IN SUFFERING.

Why does God allow suffering? — He is doing His utmost to prevent it; but man refuses to conform. Three great purposes of suffering are:

>To warn of deflection from the Law.

>To make people sick of sinning.

>To refine and spiritualise.

Through defective spiritual polarisation and concomitant failure man brings his sufferings on himself. But God, within, uses them, when we react favourably, to draw us into happier relationship with Himself.

Suffering is redemptive. To seek to remove the most potent of stimuli, without promoting a higher response, may be woeful disservice. The true healer will seek to encourage this higher response and obedience. Healing will be incidental.

ONLY ONE WAY.

There is absolutely no other healing power whatsoever in existence than SPIRIT; and no other means whereby He may heal than repentance, obedience, and increasing polarisation.

All man can do to help in the physical-mental realms is to co-operate by supplying the requisite materials, and by removal or facilitating removal, in body or mind, of whatever may be acting as a barrier in the path of the Life-giving Power.

THERE IS ONLY ONE HEALING POWER—THE LIFE FORCE WITHIN.

WHAT IS THAT FORCE?—THE SPIRIT OF GOD.

WHERE IS THAT SPIRIT?—AROUND EVERY ONE, AND WITHIN.

HOW DOES HE WORK?—BY FAITH, THROUGH REPENTANCE, AND OBEDIENCE TO LAW.

II. RIGHT THINKING

"Hear, O earth, behold, I will bring evil upon this people, EVEN THE FRUIT OF THEIR THOUGHTS because they have not hearkened unto my words, nor to my law, but rejected it."

Jeremiah VI, 19.

FOR long ages, as we reckon time, man has been evolving from his primitive origin. The natural, animal man, the first man, "is of the earth, earthy. The second man (the spiritual Self), is the Lord from Heaven." Our bodies and minds have been slowly evolved over long periods of time; "that was not first which is spiritual, but that which is natural; and afterward that which is spiritual." Their purpose is to serve as increasingly effective instruments for the expression of Spirit.

For millions of years man lived a purely animal existence. Eventually, a stage was reached when as Adamic man, "God breathed into his nostrils the breath of life." Man began, that is to say, for the first time, to be dimly and intermittently aware of some influence for GOOD, apparently apart from himself. His consciousness, at first solely physical, became, as he evolved, intellectual-physical. Gradually, and through unnumbered vicissitudes this awareness unfolded until, during the last few thousand years, the more responsive have become increasingly conscious of the Influence as a Presence. More and more rapidly, in this Epoch of Adamic experience, is consciousness evolving of this Presence as Spirit, First Cause, God; and of ourselves as spiritual beings, continuous with and part of Spirit.

SPIRITUAL PHYSICS.

Corresponding to the seven primary colours of the spectrum of physical light there are seven stages of spiritual consciousness (or "Light") , from the purely animal to the perfectly spiritual; and a positive constructive and negative destructive of every degree of each stage. In the winter "season" of the fifth, blue, of the seven stages, or "times," the spiritual first becomes the dominating factor. But until spiritual consciousness is fully developed, the conflict is ever between the higher spiritual and the lower physical-intellectual of our duality. (L. E. B.)

At the lower end of the spectrum of spiritual light are the slow, hot, long-wave, red, and infra-red vibrations, intensely destructive in the negative. It is more than coincidence that the Bolshevik flag is red, for might and feat are their driving force. Jacob, symbolizing the responsive section of humanity-Adam in the transition period from spiritual darkness to light, gave his son a coat of many colours. (L. E. B.)

At the higher end of the spectrum are the fine, short wave, purple, and ultra-violet, high vibrations, powerfully healing and constructive in the positive, of spiritual love. (They wrought more spiritually than they suspected who brought forth the purple robe for the King they were mocking.) (L. E. B.)

In the lower stages, or "Times," man is in bondage to the Law; in higher "Times," he becomes "delivered from the bondage of corruption into the glorious liberty of the children of God."

Men are at varying stages of physical and spiritual evolution, from the gigantic and animal, towards the finer more ethereal. Those at the red, long-wave, lower end of the Adamic gamut, in whom spiritual consciousness is limited to an intermittent flicker, of dense, heavy texture, and usually gross physical strength, are dependent for their prospects of recovery from disease upon the great recuperative powers innate within the natural man. These resources will be found inferior to the spiritual regenerative influence, of higher vibration, available to those at the purple end of the spectrum. *Thus a weak, physically devitalised individual, of high spiritual potentiality and polarisation, will exhibit powers of recovery far beyond those available to the less responsive.* (L. E. B.)

"JACOB'S TROUBLE."

Man is body, mind, spirit; and corresponding to this triune existence, there are three "World" orders: the physical World (order) that was, that in humanity Adamic processing merged through the Flood Epoch into the Japhetic (Gentile) Intellectual World (order) that now is; which in its turn is in an Epoch, merging into the SPIRITUAL WORLD (order) that is to be. We are in the time of "Jacobs' Trouble" — the transitional period in Adamic experience from physical intellectual to spiritual dominance. It is a period of chaos and flux, preparatory to the founding of a new age. The mass Adam is at the critical period encountered sooner or later by each individual—the winter "season" of the fifth stage, or "Time." (L. E. B.)

The significance of this principle, with all its ramifications, must be gripped, and its application studied and understood; because medical men, though not wanting in the spirit of the ideal, fail in that, lacking the spiritual PRINCIPLE, they do not comprehend its application through the Law. It matters little how high the misaligned idealism. The will to do right does not assure the deed; "nor does potentiality necessarily connote eventuality!" Not until physical and intellectual man is definitely and finally subordinated to the Spiritual, will he be able to apprehend Spiritual plan, process and purpose, and the Law through which they are expressed.

HUMAN WISDOM AND GOOD INTENTION, IN ANY SPHERE OF ACTIVITY, ARE SPIRITUALLY EFFECTIVE ONLY TO THE DEGREE OF ALIGNMENT WITH THE SPIRIT AND LAW OF GOD.

CREATIVE POWER.

Few seem to realise the power of the human mind, with its almost unlimited potentialities for evil or good. Man is a spiritual being. The Spirit that is the true You, the true Me, that was and is Christ, that is God, is all ONE. Not different spirits, but different phases of one constituent—Spirit, the great invisible Power "in Whom we live and move and have our being," of Whom both physically and spiritually we are phase manifestations. Therefore there are, latent and awaiting development within each one of us, all the resources and attributes of Spirit. The characteristic particularly distinguish-ing Spirit in the absolute, from His relative manifestations, is creative ability. And Spirit creates by thought; He thinks His ideas into materialisation. THOUGHT IS THE CREATIVE INSTRUMENT.

And since we are spiritual beings this faculty is inherent within. Whether consciously or not, all use it to greater or less extent. Negatively directed it leads to disaster and death. Positively aligned it functions constructively to well-being. Therefore the imperative necessity for right thinking, *for sooner or later, good, bad, or utterly disastrous, in ourselves, in those we love or dislike, ultimately in the world as a whole, the thoughts we hold in our minds will materialise.* In ourselves and our circumstances, individual, community, nation, world, we are what we have made ourselves; and may become what we choose to be.

PENALTIES EXACTED BY MISUSE.

"Whatsoever a man soweth that shall he also reap."

Galatians VI, 7.

Few stop to consider the destructive influence of negative thoughts. They are pregnant with ruin. They destroy not merely mental happiness and efficiency but actual physical tissue as well. Mental disharmony is reflected through sympathetic and endocrine upset as actual physical disease.

Growths, diabetes, high blood pressure and strokes, skin diseases, heart and kidney disorders, goitre, anaemia, neuritis, paralysis and other organic nervous disease, rheumatism, and rheumatoid, asthma, cancer, as well as broken homes, poverty, wretchedness, suicide, murder, insanity, war, can be and most frequently are a direct result of holding in the mind thoughts of fear, greed, hate, frustration, bitterness, resentment, self-pity, meanness, intolerance, cruelty, lust. Such calamities will cease when the mental habit responsible is reversed.

THOUGHTS ARE VIBRATORY FORCES.

Medical men are generally of strong, often powerful, personality. Many still in deflection or sense-sleep are of exceptional potentiality. Awakened and progressively polarised, they will discover in themselves a new unsuspected POWER TO HEAL, of growing effectiveness.

Meanwhile, befooled by stubborn allegiance to human physical wisdom, such men by misaligned methods and outlook, achieve incalculable harm. The mountains labour, and bring forth—*a germ*!

". . . . in whom the god of this world (human physical wisdom) hath blinded the minds of them that believe not. . . ."

The thought atmosphere in hospitals and asylums, being almost invariably unspiritual, is disconcertingly negative. Again and again trivial symptoms, or minor or major healing reactions, are misunderstood, magnified through ignorance, FEAR, tradition, and calamitous wrong treatment, *and intensified by disease and death thoughts in the minds of all concerned into chronic or fatal disorder.*

And so people often with little amiss are consigned in battalions and army corps to their graves.

IN WAR, GUIDES WHO MISLEAD THE ARMY ARE SHOT!

Such deadly thought vibrations must be stoutly withstood; and deprived of all power by realising the error, denying its strength, and triumphantly affirming and, KNOWING THE PRESENCE AND POWER OF GOOD.

WHAT WE THINK AND SPEAK OF, WE BRING INTO BEING.

Many vociferate that if they were not so worried, or poor, or sick, they could live a much happier, more spiritual life. That is partly true. But they do not grasp, and are usually reluctant to learn, that commonly it is precisely because they worry and fret that they are poverty-stricken and sick.

Our strongest mental impressions always materialise, sooner or later, in selves and surroundings. Garrulous or moaning obsession with symptoms, operations, sensations, injustices, cancer, poverty, or horrors, is not merely *advertising* that our mind is a charnel-house—it is setting time working bringing these to us. Christ blasted the fig tree, not because it did not bear figs out of season; but to demonstrate the power of negative vibration.

Never again, whatever befall, allow anything or anyone to beguile us, even for a moment, into working the Creative Power within, to our own or others' undoing.

Worry, gluttony, sex abuse, sour temper, many "fits," and much sickness and poverty, are simply BAD HABITS OF MIND. They can and must be defeated—not by fighting the negative, but by assiduously practising their positive opposites. It is mostly a matter of WILLINGNESS—willingness to have done with the negative: to make the necessary small sacrifice for the sake of GOOD.

Therefore:
1. RECOGNIZE THE ADVISABILITY.
2. MAKE UP YOUR MIND.
3. STAND PORTER AT YOUR MENTAL THRESHOLD.

Indulgence of all kinds is bondage. Spirit redeems, if we will.

If husband, wife, friend, "foe," or acquaintance, be acting unkindly or worse, do not let that perturb. Not what happens, nor what is said about or to us can hurt, but ONLY OUR WRONG REACTION THERETO.

We are seldom responsible for the thoughts or actions of others—we are for our own! Therefore see that, whatever goes on outside us, inside is, never, anything but quiet good humour, sweetness, wise tolerance, patience, tact, imperturbable confidence, and love.

GOD'S POWER WORKS THROUGH OUR FAITH, therefore set that POWER to work by warm FAITH. There is NOTHING it cannot heal in time: nagging, drunkenness, selfishness, vice, MUST give way, if you persevere.

So, now, if in the past you have unthinkingly misdirected this vast force, BEGIN, AT. ONCE, TO USE IT ARIGHT. AND HAVING BEGUN—KEEP IT UP. You will be thrilled, and humbled, and uplifted as you see the results. Life will be LIFE INDEED.

CONSIDER THE LILLIES.

When the Bible says "Your bodies are the temple of God's Spirit" it is not making a religious assertion merely, it is stating a profound scientific truth.

Everyone knows by experience that cuts will heal in a week or two; and that if they do not, something must be preventing them.

Cuts do not heal accidentally or automatically, but in response to a regenerative process set in operation and controlled by an Inner Directive Intelligence—the Spirit of God—working through the subconscious mind.

The Power that heals a cut or mends a fracture is the same that deals with a toxic condition or psychological disorder. Its Nature is what Christ showed it to be—infinitely loving and perfectly patient, with one great passion and purpose for each of His human children: our highest good.

No unhealthy condition however advanced or depraved is ultimately beyond the redemptive effect of God's Love.

If then we have some disease, whether in body, mind, soul, or estate, not being healed, it is not because the Spirit within has passed us by, or is no longer trying to mend our hurts; but usually because SOMETHING IS PREVENTING HIM ACHIEVING HIS PURPOSE.

5. The Part Man Must Play

"Repent, and turn yourselves from all your transgressions; so iniquity shall not be your ruin. Cast away from you all your transgressions, whereby ye have transgressed; AND MAKE YOU A NEW HEART AND A NEW SPIRIT: for why will ye die, O house of Israel'? For I have no pleasure in the death of him that saith the Lord God: Wherefore turn yourselves, and live ye."

Ezekiel XVIII, 30.

THE causes of Disease, it has been postulated, are:
1. PRIMARY.
    — PSYCHOLOGICAL:
        (a) Wrong Mental and, Emotional Tensions, or thoughts.
        (b) Wrong impressions, beliefs, suggestions, or ideas in the conscious or subconscious mind.
    — PHYSICAL:
        (a) Misuse of foods.
        (b) Faulty general habits.

2. SECONDARY.
    — Toxic.
    — Economic.
    — "Accidental."
    — Environmental.

THERE are two main Types of Healing God uses for mending man's hurts...

I. PHYSICAL: THE NATURAL REGENERATIVE PROCESS, coming into operation, more or less effectively according to circumstances, when the causes are corrected — whereby the degenerative disease process is arrested and converted into a regenerative healing process. Our object being to heal, we shall have to remember three things. We must:

   (A) **Correct the Causes** — both Primary and Secondary; for we can hardly expect the Power within to heal while causes are allowed to continue. This is frequently one of the worst of our difficulties, since, while few would not willingly part with their symptoms, many would die a dozen times over (and quite likely have), rather than give up the causes.

   (B) **Supply Deficiencies, and Promote Elimination of Waste** — where such is needed; for not even Nature can reconstruct without materials, or heavily hampered by rubbish.

   (C) **Co-operate with Nature's Curative Efforts** — interfering with which has become the great secondary cause of disease.

II. MENTAL AND SPIRITUAL, whereby the Natural Process can be fortified and expedited, to the degree of spiritual receptivity and response

6. Correcting Psychological Causes

"My son, give attention to my words; incline your ear to my sayings. Do not let them depart from your eyes; keep them in the midst of your heart; for they are life to those who find them, and health to all their flesh."

Proverbs IV, 20-22.

I. WRONG MENTAL AND EMOTIONAL THOUGHTS

These are the Negative destructive mental reactions characteristic of the lower animal nature with its physical consciousness. While perfectly Natural, they were developed as protective reactions during the long ages of physical evolving. Having served their purpose they must be rigorously set aside, for they are directly opposed to the developing Positive constructive attributes of the higher angelic nature, with its spiritual consciousness.

Animal characteristics and spiritual attributes are *mutually antagonistic*; they represent the negative and positive of the Spirit of Life.

In only one way can the natural-man characteristics be overcome — never by fighting them, but by turning from them resolutely, and steadfastly cultivating their positive opposites.

Not only is continued development possible on no other terms; but progress already achieved will be sacrificed through neglecting to measure up to new spiritual standards.

DON'T FIGHT DISEASE, but PRACTICE GOOD HEALTH.

Claim it, think it, feel it, believe in it, and dare to manifest it. That is what brings it about.

"Resist not evil; but overcome evil with Good." *If you wish to become good, be good; if you wish to become well, begin immediately, to BE WELL.*

Fear and Disease-consciousness, and that barbaric embodiment of them both, *maternal solicitude,* are among the greatest of all causes of disease; and if disease is to go from our bodies, we *must* let it go from our minds.

After all, man is a spiritual being, part of and continuous with the Universal Life Spirit, whose perfect attributes are those, of the Radiant, Inner, True SELF. Good health, happiness, safety, prosperity, are appurtenances of the spiritual state; and can be attained in no other way.

GLAND INFLUENCE AND CONTROL.

There exists in our body a chain of internal secreting glands, interdependent, producing highly complex substances profoundly influencing bodily structure and functioning. These glands, thyroid, pituitary, ovaries, testicles, prostate, suprarenals, parathyroids, are exceedingly sensitive to emotional stimulus.

For instance, through acute fear an individual may become blanched, pulseless, and unable to move. The pallor and rapid pulse are caused by 'the constricting effect, upon the skin capillary blood vessels, of thyroid and suprarenal secretion, discharged into the circulation by the fear stimulus; and by excitation of relevant nerve control. The blood vessels of the stomach and intestines are similarly affected; deprivation of the supply of blood essential to the elaboration of digestive fluids, completely prevents digestion. A meal taken shortly before a fright or shock may be vomited many hours later, completely undigested. This is why worry, which is fear, and mental tension generally, cause so much indigestion. Blanching of mucous membrane through emotional tension predisposes to auto-digestion, and formation of gastric and duodenal ulcers, the majority of which arise in this way. The remainder are almost all due to misuse of food.

SOME EFFECTS OF DISTURBANCE.

Interference with functioning of any internal secreting gland disturbs all the others, particularly when the body is in a toxic condition. Poisons of many kinds depress or exaggerate activity of glands, and may damage and even destroy their delicate structure. Food, intestinal, drug, and bacterial poisons are highly deleterious; and perverted secretion itself becomes toxic.

The parathyroid and thyroid glands are concerned continuously with detoxication. The pituitary, influences growth, metabolism, sex functioning and reproduction. The ovaries regulate development, menstruation, and pregnancy. The male sex glands are intimately engaged with energy and vital control. The suprarenals influence arterial tension and blood pressure. The functions of all glands are inextricably bound up together, and interact. They may wreck or be wrecked by all kinds of activities; and affect, and are directly affected by, thought.

Diabetes and goitre are perversions of structure or function occasioned by fear or other emotion; and, or, by auto-intoxication, as well as deficiency.

Acromegaly develops through pituitary malfunctioning, caused by fear or other upset. Obesity of a special type results from pituitary disorder; and ranks as one of the toxic-deficiency effects.

Prostatic enlargement is frequently caused by sexual over-excitement, with local congestion and toxic accumulation, Naturally, poisons tend to accumulate wherever circulation is interfered with. This partly explains why cancer develops in the site of old inflammations or scars.

Sterility, haemorrhages, abortions, and still births can be caused by glandular aberration; due to negative emotion, acute or chronic poisoning, or mineral or vitamin deficiency.

Fibroid growths are toxic in origin, and often associated with sex mismanagement and repression.

Stimulation of suprarenal secretion by worry or fret, causes raised arterial tension, high blood pressure, heart and kidney disease, and strokes; so does the "carbon clogging" of Stone, resulting from gluttony.

Resentment and bitterness pervert internal secretion; and some of the most formidable skin disorders, such as "seborrheic dermatitis," may be caused in this way; the skin becoming acutely inflamed by the intensely irritant secretions eliminated.

Many acute illnesses are simply evidence of elimination, through one or other of the regular or subsidiary channels, of effete matter resulting from violent emotion.

Jealousy causes neuritis and rheumatism; meanness desiccates; rage will cause acute catarrhal disorder; irritability may set up tonsillitis; gluttony and laziness produce obesity, gall stones, constipation, and cancer.

Remember, the subconscious mind can imitate or elaborate any disorder; and while Fear destroys; Confidence reconstructs.

THE VALLEY OF DECISION.

It is as if God, at the back of us, puts at our disposal potentially unlimited power and the means to set it to work; and then leaves it to us, by rightful exercise of our will, to learn to control it aright.

Not merely once in our life, but day by day, hour by hour, moment by moment, we are compelled to make a choice:

Which shall it be—

The destructive, degenerative, NEGATIVE disease producing Wrong Thoughts, the NATURAL, ANIMAL-MAN CHARACTERISTICS? or the constructive, regenerative, POSITIVE, health maintaining, Right Thoughts, the SPIRITUAL, HIGHER-SELF ATTRIBUTES?

The two choices lead in opposite directions—the former downwards, through sickness, unhappiness, poverty, to disease, misery, disaster, destruction, despair. The latter leads upwards to LIGHT and LIFE, to health, and happiness, and general well-being, of body, mind, soul and estate, for ourselves, for those we love, and all we come in contact with; in fact, for the world at large.

"I WILL BRING EVIL..."

Wrong Thoughts are, by far, the greatest of all causes of disease. For instance:

FEAR—of anything, past, present, or future, however impossible or unlikely. Fear of death; fear of disease; fear of poverty; fear of what others may say.

WORRY—its twin brother; the child of ignorance and unbelief: "For if GOD be for us, who can be against us?"

ANXIETY—which can exist no more than either of the preceding in the presence of faith. The little sneaking Doubt that short circuits Spiritual power. It was unbelief that prevented Jesus Christ from doing His mighty works in Nazareth. Its effect is exactly the same today.

DOUBT — the barrier that arises from the intellect — "Why this is Jesus, the carpenter's son."

RESENTMENT — against life, or fate; or something we have suffered at the hands of others; or that has been said, or that we imagine has been or might have been said about us.

SELF-PITY — that hateful, hellish, and inexcusable pandering to weakness, of the repressed undeveloped animal consciousness.

SELFISHNESS — self-centredness having yet to learn that none can find life except those who have lost it for Christ's sake.

THOUGHTS OF WEAKNESS — inferiority, depression, ineffectiveness, shortage or limitation of any kind, while the true US is Spirit — potential might, perfection, and power incarnate.

GRIEF — so often prolonged into selfish yielding to the destructive influences of weakness, resentment, and self-pity; a barbarous denial of the implications of Christ's resurrection.

CRAVING FOR SYMPATHY — that relic of infantile mentality.

INDIFFERENCE — to the rights and sufferings of others.

BAD-TEMPER — and its homologues; bitterness, irritability, touchiness, vindictiveness, impatience, uncharitableness, and intolerance, that exact such a frightful toll in misery of body and mind.

DISCONTENT — that saps all the joy of life.

- SELF-INDULGENCE—seeing that self-restraint is the price of self-respect.
- PRIDE, VANITY, JEALOUSY, MEANNESS, CRUELTY, SLOTH, GREED—Avarice, love of money, "THE ROOT OF ALL EVIL."
- GLUTTONY—one of the hardest to subdue.
- LUST—the very blight of life. Sex wastage in married or single is not simply unspiritual, it is definitely anti-spiritual. The sex appetite is for many the hardest of all to subdue; but, like a craving for alcohol, tobacco, or other corrosives, will leave us as soon as we really wish. Simply MAKE UP YOUR MIND once and for all, that now and for ever, you will exhibit only the indwelling, purity and sweetness of the inner true spiritual SELF.

A small struggle—truly a minor one—to exercise volition constructively. The reason for failure is ape-self reluctance to yield to the angel-SELF. But the Spirit within WILL redeem, if we acquiesce.

"QUIETNESS AND CONFIDENCE SHALL BE THY STRENGTH."

No individual can indefinitely be healthier than his thoughts; nor his body than the cells it consists of. Neither can any nation be healthier than its thoughts; nor its body than the people composing it. It is a fear-ridden and sin-sick world, which, like the individuals that compose it, can be healed only through love of God expressing in perfect obedience to His Law. Fear—the medical system is built up on, thrives upon, inculcates, and couldn't exist without, fear. Fear of acute illness—which is Nature's method of cure. Fear of chronic disease, which seldom exists if we comply with the requirements of health. People proclaim their faith in God; but worry is fear and "FEAR IS FAITH IN EVIL" WHICH IS THE DEAD OPPOSITE OF FAITH IN GOOD WHICH IS FAITH IN GOD.

There are not two powers. Evil—the devil—is merely inverted GOOD. Only when GOOD is disobeyed or misapplied does evil result. There is no power in evil except such as we concede it; and no evil at all if we are conscious only of GOOD.

"THE KINGDOM OF GOOD IS WITHIN."

RIGHT THOUGHTS are, by far, the greatest of all human influences that heal.

FAITH—the developing faculty of the higher spiritual man. Faith, the quiet, rejoicing assurance that the Power behind all these material-seeming appearances is only and always GOOD.

CONFIDENCE—the practical expression of faith.

CERTAINTY—fruit of developing consciousness that dispels misgiving.

SELF-FORGETFULNESS—finding in service that which was fruitlessly sought in indulgence.

EXULTATION IN STRENGTH—because God is our Father, and is the rewarder of them that diligently seek Him.

HAPPINESS—because we open our hearts to God's revelation of Himself in Christ, and in Us.

COMPASSION—Love's partner, the harbinger of healing.

SWEET-TEMPER—gentleness, patience, charitableness, tolerance, long-suffering; the very soothing balm.

CONSIDERATION—for the sufferings and rights of others that

will not let us rest while there is one sick, one poor, or one oppressed.

CONTENTMENT — because Christ promised "If a man love me, he will keep my commandments; and my Father will love him, and we will come unto him, and make our abode with him."

SELF-CONTROL — for thus do we keep His commandments.

HUMILITY, GENEROSITY, FRANKNESS, ENERGY, IMPERTURBABILITY.

SELF-SACRIFICE — recognizing "money" for what it should be, a trust-machinery for the distribution of goods and services.

TEMPERANCE — the key to right use and enjoyment.

PURITY — our realisation of the Divine.

LOVE — the VERY HIGHEST ATTRIBUTE OF GOD; THE MOST POWERFUL HEALING VIBRATION; the VERY ESSENCE OF LIFE.

"THOU WILT KEEP HIM IN PERFECT PEACE WHOSE MIND IS STAYED ON THEE."

People often protest intellectual difficulty; but spiritual difficulties are seldom intellectual, they are almost invariably moral. It is our *heart* God wants, not merely our head.

Have you finally made your choice? You will follow an increasingly chequered career till you do! Affirmations are good. The POWER is there; and it works through our faith. But we can learn to develop latent potentiality by practice alone. *It is actions that count, not what we say we believe.* Actions must be aligned to spiritually instructed perception. No man wins championships by sitting on the side line and affirming potentiality. Nor does he succeed at the first attempt. NO! Affirm the potentiality, then set out in patience, cheerfulness, determination and perseverance to put it to the proof.

And the justification? — that we *are* spiritual beings, one with the Lord Jesus Christ and God our Father; that God IS what Christ showed Him to be, and therefore the power IS IN US, if we turn in complete surrender to Him, that will unfailingly honour our faith.

PRACTISE THE PRESENCE OF GOD.

WE MUST deal with the "old Adam." Crucify him, St Paul advises. Turn from him always and instantly; learn and practise continuously so to live in the higher consciousness of our true Spiritual Self that the attributes of the Spirit are manifest in every thought and action. No life for weaklings! We shall find our highest qualities tested to their utmost limit; and, it may be, far beyond. But what can any man ask better of life than an almost impossible task and an absolutely invincible POWER!

We are offered glorious, magnificent, thrilling LIFE! "Liberation from the bondage of corruption into the glorious liberty of the children of God."

"PERFECT LOVE CASTETH OUT FEAR."

Well! The choice lies before YOU. Which shall it be? Selfishness, or self-sacrifice? Misery, or happiness? Poverty, or wealth? Sickness, or health? Bondage, or freedom? Darkness, or light? Evil, or Good?

You can't have it both ways. You MUST make a choice.

Do NOT say, "I'll try" — that is merely postponing the decision we have always shirked.

Do not say, "I'm going to"—tomorrow never comes. The decision MUST be made NOW. There are only two possible answers. No middle course. Which shall it be?

YES? . . . . or . . . . NO. One little step in faith, from the apparent comparative security of our physical foundation into the unknown—but our foot will come down on rock, and that ROCK is CHRIST.

II. WRONG IDEAS IN THE SUBCONSCIOUS MIND

Everyone knows that the Conscious Mind controls voluntary function; but it is not so generally recognized that the Subconscious Mind controls involuntary function.

The mind may be likened roughly to a tree, having a conscious visible part above ground, as it were; and a subconscious, invisible, underground.

The Conscious Mind is the critical, reasoning part of our mental make-up; it selects, decides, and discriminates. The Subconscious Mind is non-critical, executive; it acts upon, and carries out to the limit of ability, right or wrong, without attempting to criticise, the impressions, beliefs, suggestions, or ideas implanted into it, whether through the operation of the Conscious Mind, without its intervention, even, maybe, despite disapproval.

And, since the Subconscious Mind controls involuntary functioning,

BEWARE THE IDEA IT IS WORKING UPON.

THE SUBCONSCIOUS TRAP.

The Subconscious Mind is immensely impressionable; particularly so where (as in childhood), the conscious critical faculty is under-developed; or where for any reason, such for example as debility or preoccupation, it is temporarily in abeyance.

In case after case, the outward evidences of disease are surface signs of some fear or belief imprinted upon the infant subconscious, and deepened by passage of time.

Suggestions of weakness or inferiority thoughtlessly or cruelly implanted in a child's subconscious before the critical faculty is sufficiently grown to be a protection, bear ruinous fruit. Children are twanged like piano wires by the thought vibrations around. In homes where selfish passions hold sway, havoc is wrought; and may still be working years later.

A "difficult" child is usually reacting to dread of unwantedness. All crave love and appreciation. Indifference, or menace to self-esteem, evoke, in the under-evolved, negative efforts to compensate.

Much adult illness is a clumsy maladjustment to ill-usage, fancied or real. To elicit a constructive link-up will often demand inexhaustible patience.

Sickness sensitises; and hyperacute perception, craving encouragement, intuitively discerns attendants' subconscious convictions, even disguised. The forebodings of fearful minds, heedlessly reinforced or confirmed, can become lifelong handicaps; but the high vibrations of faith and peace are balm to sick souls. To impress the subconscious mind with death thoughts is equivalent to signing the death warrant. Hope or faith may provide a reprieve.

Expectation of occurrence, or recurrence, of any disorder contrives subconscious fulfilment.

Beliefs in the reality or inevitability of disease, or in the power of the material physical to limit or dominate, confer upon it such powers.

Subconsciously fashioned disease is a favourite artifice of the timid, slothful, or selfish, to evade obligation, protest at "misfortune," or focus sympathy and attention.

"Be careful what you want, for you are sure to get it." So reads a caption; and fulfilment of subconscious wish explains many a "mysterious" tragedy, event, mishap, achievement, or stroke of good fortune. Innumerable diseases and "accidents," subconsciously engineered, are plausible substitutes for deliberate suicide.

"Forgetting" shameful or unworthy actions or reactions is useless, and worse. It is the mechanism whereby guilty or disturbing memories are pushed out of consciousness. But the subconscious never forgets; and, there, the old bane works unrestricted, and tears body and soul into shreds.

Buried repressions of every description must be dug up, faced, and sensibly re-adjusted. Mostly, they aren't far down!

Unrealised fears of misunderstood sex tensions, promptings, or cravings, cause oceans of misery. So out with those peccadilloes into the light of day! They are characteristics of the animal nature; and it is the FEAR, not past acts or shortcomings, that harms. Wrong of all kinds, sincerely repented, is not merely forgiven—the slate is wiped clean.

When the conscience-stricken king called anxiously into the noisome den, to Daniel beset on all sides by ravening beast (forces): "Is the God, whom thou servest continually, able to deliver thee from the lions?"—the prophet, serene in pure consciousness of sweet spiritual PRESENCE was able to cry . . .

"O king, live for ever! My God hath sent His angel, and hath shut the lions' mouths, and they have not hurt me."

Daniel VI, 21.

The subconscious mind will go on creating disease until the motivating idea, completely mistaken or seemingly justified, is reversed. This may be accomplished in several ways; for example:

1. *By practising the positive opposite*: that is, by changing, voluntarily, the mental outlook and habit of mind; and always assiduously practising positive thoughts.
2. *By suggestion*: repeating, to oneself or another, affirmations of health and well-being until, from sheer repetition, the subconscious mind is impressed.
3. *By positive superimposure*: by one of sufficiently powerful personality and conviction forcibly replacing a disease belief with a new and more powerful mental health belief.

But the best and quickest way—a way Christ habitually employed—is (in those of adequate consciousness or potentiality) to induce and inspire, through compassion and love, and intensity of pellucid perception, overwhelming subconscious (and so presently conscious) recognition of spiritual unity, wholeness, perfection.

This method can be perfected only, as the Lord Jesus put it, "by prayer and fasting"—and then, subject to relativity. Final at-one-ment of self, through spiritual SELF, with the Divine PRESENCE "who is above all, and through all, and IN you ALL," must be our goal; for through us, as progress is made, the afflicted will be lifted by SPIRIT above the mental and physical illusory planes where sickness and sin occur.

7. Correcting Physical Causes

"And God said, Behold, I have given you every herb bearing seed, . . . and every tree, in the which is the fruit of a tree yielding seed; to you it shall be for food."

Genesis I, 29.

I. MISUSE OF FOODS

Fruits, vegetables, nuts, and whole grains were the food intended for Adamic man. So long as he kept to this diet, man lived nigh a thousand years. Not till the time of Noah did he revert to pre-Adamic cravings for meat; and invent strong drink. When he did, the length of his days was reduced to one hundred and twenty years. With the advent of food-fouling methods, man's span fell to as little as forty years. With hygiene improved, and wiser counsels in feeding, the length of man's days is gradually growing again. With developing consciousness, and better observance of cosmic law, man's sojourn on earth will rapidly lengthen once more.

People often say "I don't see how diet can cure disease." The answer of course is, it cannot. But wrong feeding can and does cause much disease; and right feeding removes from the path of the Life-giving Power one of the conditions that act as a barrier.

COMMONSENSE FOODS, NOT "DIET."

There are many who say it does not matter what we eat; but a sound building cannot be constructed of defective materials, and since the body is built of what we put into it, better surely use good foods than bad. No one who planted a tree in the hope of enjoying the fruits would think of planting it in soil known to be impoverished and where no sunlight came.

Then why treat our bodies so?

Wrong feeding might almost be defined as living upon the conventional diet. Not even the most ardent "scientist" would maintain that food is still food *after* it has passed through the body—neither is most of it after it has passed through the machines of the manufacturers.

"Primitive men and animals, living on natural, un-manipulated food, are free from indigestion, free from constipation, free from auto-intoxication, free from dental decay, and FREE FROM CANCER. Where food is natural and primitive, these troubles are seldom if ever encountered. Where food is 'scientifically' improved, refined, and adulterated, dental decay, pyorrhoea, indigestion, constipation, autointoxication, appendicitis, colitis, diabetes AND CANCER are wide-spread."

—J. Ellis Barker (1870-1948), British naturopath.

THE FOOD RAMP.

Food-faking is perpetrated not to increase nutritive value, which is always dangerously reduced thereby, but with the unmoral object of pandering to perverted taste, and exploiting the people's need. Money, profit, and greed are enthroned, not the Kingdom of God and His righteousness.

Most people live, either from choice or necessity, on cheap, processed, de-vitalised. foods. *But dead foods cannot support life or good health.* Ignorance of this truth cost the great Captain Scott and his fellow-explorers their lives. It has cost the lives, health, and happiness of millions of others since; and continues to levy toll.

The ideal diet does not exist. Hardly one single article of food but is deficient, denatured, or doped. So savage and pitiless is exploitation that to large numbers an adequate diet is out of reach altogether. In a country that could be carpeted a foot deep in vegetables and fruit, these primary essentials are always in short supply. Prices are forced up on any excuse until necessities of most kinds become rich men's luxuries.

Genuine wholemeal has been hard to get: the death-dealing white flour pays better. Raw sugar is scarce because plant is designed to produce white. Contaminated milk is pasteurised in order to free it from infection rather than organise clean and wholesome supplies.

At the dictates of an iniquitous distributing system, we are forced to export our best food, and content ourselves with second or third grade at exorbitant prices. We market "excess" in foreign countries, while our own people go short.

SCATTY INDIFFERENCE.

The heedless abuse of foods in our schools, hospitals, boarding houses, hotels, Government Institutions, and worst of all in our homes, exemplifies unteachableness. Health camps are monuments not to King George the Fifth, but to blindness and apathy. The proper place for health camps is in the homes of the people.

THE "APE'S" FINAL FLING.

In a dying world order dedicated to grab instead of to service, the major food crimes are connected with: PRODUCTION, PRESERVATION, PREPARATION, DISTRIBUTION, CONSUMPTION.

PRODUCTION OFFENCES include deforestation; shallow cultivation; failure to observe orderly rotation and fallow periods; neglect of correct fertilisation; forcing with artificial fertilisers and manures; exploiting and exporting the mineral wealth of the soil, exhausting humus and mineral content; spraying with dangerous poisons; disposal of sewage into rivers and sea.

Among the consequences are vitamin and mineral deficiency, and toxic accumulation; soil depletion and erosion; pests; floods; dust storms; droughts; human and stock disease; mental and physical decadence and decay; and, in the words of Thomas Stone (1879-1959), "universal race suicide."

PRESERVATION, like production, is inspired primarily by profit, not service. Live foods do not keep well; so the obvious thing is to kill them. This is done by refining and processing. Few have troubled that, in so doing, foods are robbed of the essential life-elements.

REFINED FOODS ARE DEAD FOODS; AND DEAD FOODS ARE DEATH-DEALING.

Most of the foods in popular favour are dead. The penalties involved are fantastic. To point out the peril incurs derision and scorn.

We are plundered, despoiled, and robbed; and we ourselves are the thieves.

SUICIDAL IMBECILITY.

There would be a riot if, even inadvertently, second-grade benzine were put in our cars; but we indignantly reject the first-grade fuels provided by the Designer for our own infinitely more highly evolved and specialised vehicles, and replenish our tanks with corrosives.

Foods persistently man-handled are often useless, and by no means infrequently dangerous; but of late years the menace has grown still more portentous by the addition as preservative, colouring, and flavouring agents, of a variety of murderous chemicals. So great has this evil grown that in most households NOT ONE ITEM OF FOOD IS CONSUMED THAT IS POISON FREE.

Some of the drugs employed are known to be cancer-producing; all are admittedly harmful; but who can ever compute the full extent of their ravages!

Alum, arsenic, antimony, benzoic acid and benzoates, boracic acid and borax, salicylic acid and salicylates; sulphur, sulphuric acid, sulphurous acid, sulphates, sulphites; chlorine, chlorides, chlorates, hypochlorites; spirits of wine; fluorides; formalin; lead, tin, copper, aluminium, zinc; mercury; a great variety of aniline dyes, and coal tar derivatives generally; and perhaps worst of all an increasing range of synthetic atrocities. All these are added to food.

"WE ARE BOMBARDED WITH CHEMICALS AND POISONS IN SMALL QUANTITIES AND AT ALL MEALS. THE QUANTITY TAKEN AT ANY ONE TIME MAY BE HARMLESS; BUT THE CUMULATIVE EFFECT SPELLS CATASTROPHE"

— thus a famous public analyst.

In aniline works in Belgium it was found that cancer of the bladder occurred in operatives as long as thirty years after a period of work as short as three months. Yet aniline dyes are taken daily in food! [Aniline is toxic to humans but the more carcinogenic agent in the dye industry was later thought to be 1-naphthylamine, S.A.H.B.]

Arsenic, a known cancer producer, gains entrance to our bodies in a great many ways; and is a most favoured ingredient of ointments, "tonics," and "medicines."

Butter, cream, margarine, bacon, sausages, pies, and meat and fish pastes, contain boric acid, borax, salicylic acid, and other preservatives, besides colouring and flavouring agents. There is no real check on quantities used. As much as 140 grains per pound of boric acid has been found by analysis in marketed butter; and as high as 110 grains in sausages, and meat and fish pastes.

So also with milk. Some of the mysterious infant disorders are due to chemical poisoning.

Meat, even that sold as "fresh," is similarly mishandled; though with different poisons. Some of the newer chemicals have been found to deodorise (though without arresting the putrefactive process and production of ptomaines). This enables bad meat to be canned, and made into sausages. Hence "Ptomain" poisoning. "Fresh" fish is also "dipped" in poisonous preservatives.

Flour, shorn of its protective vitamin and mineral health elements, is bleached with nitrous gases; and bread has, added, gypsum, acid phosphates, and other "improvers."

Beer and wine barrels have been sulphured. Temperance beverages such as ginger beer, lime juice, etc., often contain salicylic and benzoic acids. So also do wines. Seven grains per pint is the usual amount; but much more is sometimes found.

Dried fruits are de-hydrated with caustics and sulphites. It is practically impossible to obtain genuine sun-dried fruits. Fresh fruits are dangerous through poisonous sprays.

Of the horrors sold as "essences," or added to sweets and coloured drinks, a heavy indictment will one day be penned.

THERE IS NOT ONE SINGLE ITEM OF FOOD IN MOST HOMES THAT IS NOT EITHER DEFICIENT, DENATURED, OR DOPED; OFTEN ALL THREE.

Disastrous ill-health, and the grosser forms of disease result; and no useful purpose is served, though "interests" are duly respected; and further proof furnished that "love of money is the root of all evil."

"Food has nothing whatever to do with it," the self-styled cancer "expert" mechanically repeats—and cannot be told, because he does not want to be told. He is only too shrewdly aware that a single well-placed torpedo may blow up the medical ship.

IN PREPARATION OF FOODS more iniquities are committed. Heat, and chemicals of all kinds such as soda and salt, modify or even destroy vitamin and mineral content. The days of boiling peeled vegetables to rags in gallons of water, and throwing down the sink what minerals are left after prolonged chemical action with soda and salt (to say nothing of aluminium and antimony) are by no means yet over. It would puzzle a rat to extract nourishment from the watery debris remaining.

The boarding-school diet of meat, sausage, curry, hash, white bread, refined cereals, tea, and mass-production jam, has one advantage over the similar fare served in most hospitals—those condemned to subsist on it get plenty of exercise. Both have the orthodox financial "virtue" of cheapness; and both sow the seeds of disease.

The tubercle bacillus is conveniently debited with the high incidence of Tuberculosis among nurses in hospitals; thus exonerating the bad food and unhealthy living conditions really responsible.

Twice cooking and re-hashing foods destroys their food value. Cooking should be resorted to as seldom as possible. Simplicity should be the keynote, frugality the watchword. The real purpose of food is to nourish and sustain—to satisfy hunger, NOT appetite, which is often insatiable.

DISTRIBUTION has become so lop-sided that, all over the world, production is being artificially restricted and supplies deliberately destroyed while multitudes are actually starving to death. There is one great physical reason for this: fiendish abuse, by a ruthless and diabolical monopoly, of control of THE PEOPLE'S credit and currency.

CONSUMPTION will be examined under the title of RIGHT FEEDING.

The main essentials of RIGHT FEEDING are: MODERATION, WISE CHOICE, and SENSIBLE COMBINATION.

MODERATION means eating only what is required by the body for maintenance of energy, heat and growth, and repair of tissue wastage. Gluttony is one of the "seven deadly sins"—the other six are Pride, Lust, Anger, Usury, Jealousy, Sloth.

Far less food is needed than is popularly supposed. Much of the excess is consumed under the misapprehension that food is the only source of energy, heat, and strength. But to leave out of account as a source of vitality the Spirit who is our Life Force is to identify ourselves with those responsible for the calorie absurdities. To load the system with food it does not require and cannot use is to dissipate energy in coping with overplus. Strength is reduced, not increased; and storage and eliminative mechanism, taxed beyond capacity, become clogged and blocked with masses of waste. The body may struggle on, but such burdens will beat it down.

The body is not an inanimate machine, and can safely survive, and is often better for, prolonged periods with little or no food at all. While as for feeding the acutely ill—it is a further remarkable commentary upon human intelligence that, with all his boasted wisdom, man should be the only animal that hasn't enough sense to stop eating when he is sick.

WISE CHOICE is relying upon the natural foods, as nearly as possible in the form in which they occur, instead of the refined and adulterated substitutes man has devised for the profit he can get out of them.

A good diet should consist, to an extent of about eighty per cent, of vegetables and fruits; the remaining foodstuffs together comprising the other twenty per cent. Eat the whole range, a large proportion raw; each contains something the others lack. Eat, or at least use, the skins and outer coverings whenever you can; much of the vitamin and mineral content is stored therein or thereunder, and heavy penalties have been provided for rejection.

THE REAL CAUSE OF POLIOMYELITIS.

"INFANTILE PARALYSIS" (Poliomyelitis) is a deficiency disease due to lack of Vitamin B1 (thiamine). [Polio is now known to be associated with chemical pesticides such as lead arsenate and DDT—see *Virus Mania*, 2021, S.A.H.B.]

Sir Robert McCarrison, while dietetic investigator to the Indian Government, published among many others the following significant discoveries:

1. Animals deprived of Vitamin B eventually become paralysed.
2. In animals with just enough Vitamin B to avoid disaster, paralysis may be precipitated by all sorts of influences.
3. The danger, from Vitamin B deficiency, is intensified in proportion as the rest of the diet is badly unbalanced.

Because modern food wreckers remove from whole grains the husk and germ which is its most important source, most diets are badly deficient, many dangerously so, in Vitamin B.

This deficiency is the more serious because the rest of the diet is so badly unbalanced.

It is a fact that a considerable section of the people live on the edge of a paralytic breakdown, due to deficiency of Vitamin B.

Paralysis occurs most frequently in **children** because:
1. Growing children need more Vitamin B than adults, and are more susceptible than adults to the effects of deficiency (McCarrison).
2. They often eat more rubbish than adults.
3. [They are more sensitive to some neurological toxins, S.A.H.B.]

Paralysis occurs most commonly in **summer** because:
1. Increased consumption in hot (and holiday) weather of ice-creams, coloured drinks, and refined starchy and sugary rubbish exaggerates dietary unbalance, and increases toxic accumulation.

2. Hot weather, plus sudden changes of temperature, sets up fermentation of toxic waste, with fever, and development, from cell-microzyma, of bacteria.
3. [The timing of when pesticides such as DDT were being sprayed in the environment, S.A.H.B.]

Paralysis occurs in "**epidemics**" because:

With so many Vitamin B deficient, highly toxic individuals living almost exactly alike, those nearest a breakdown naturally exhibit similar reactions under similar conditions. [Now recognized to be the simultaneous exposure to chemical environmental toxins, S.A.H.B.]

And remember:

1. The periodicity of disease.
2. All cases of paralysis are not polio-myelitis.
3. Bacteria, or microzyma, having developed, can disseminate; but the bug-hunters are in for a protracted chase!

The feverish stage being an Acute Illness, should, like any other Healing Crisis, be met by Fasting and Eliminative treatment; and the deficiency of Vitamin B made good by means of Marmite and bran-water in quantity. [Along with high-dose Vitamin C treatment, S.A.H.B.]

Distemper in dogs is the same disease, due to similar causes; and the same treatment succeeds.

"SUMMER DIARRHOEA" [A condition that essentially disappeared in first world countries by the middle of the 20th century, S.A.H.B.] is Nature's way of ridding bodies of the extra toxic matter introduced during hot weather.

WHY SPOIL OUR FOODS?

Bodily functions are carried on in an alkaline medium; and anything that interferes with the alkaline balance predisposes to disease. The acid waste resulting from metabolism of the acid-forming foods needs alkaline minerals for neutralisation and complete elimination; otherwise it collects and corrodes. Any excess of acid-forming foods in the diet, or deficiency of the alkaline, mineral bearing elements, tends to disturb the alkaline balance; great discrepancy leads to chronic acid-poisoning, or ACIDOSIS, referred to elsewhere.

So to feed, or to maltreat foods, as to reduce mineral intake below the minimum essential to health, is exactly what most people do; and are badly fooled, both by the gradualness of the degenerative disease process; and by the befuddlement of the germ-obsessed, when confronted with admonitory symptoms.

PROTECTIVE FOODS.

Fruits, vegetables, milk, and the husk and germ of whole grains are the great alkaline, acid neutralisers and eliminators. They are the natural protective foods. Shortage of these leads to acid accumulation, gradual deterioration both mental and physical, eventual breakdown, and final decrepitude. Replenishment stimulates renewed activity. This is why people who have long been subsisting on a diet defective in essentials, and who in consequence evince appropriate signs of decay, exhibit, when introduced to healthier foods, numerous evidences of excretory activity, culminating sooner or later in a healing reaction or "crisis."

Hearty eaters are sometimes dismayed for a while at the wide divergence between inclination and need; but, with cultivation, abstemiousness becomes second nature.

The advantages of a low protein diet have been so frequently demonstrated as to need no further argument.

Very little meat is required; indeed, the work of Chittenden goes to show, and experience seems to confirm, that animal proteins are unnecessary. The body soon learns to do better without. "Second-hand proteins," Thomson calls them. A Clydesdale stallion is a mountain of muscle; but he doesn't eat meat, fish, or eggs.

Dairy products and nuts provide us with protein and fat; but unsaturated fats such as olive oil are vitally important. OLIVE OIL is an invaluable anti-acid, a de-hydrator of water-logged tissues. It is Nature's marvellous anti-toxin, protector, and physical saviour.

The principal starchy foods are potatoes, whole grains, and whole-meal. These again must be used in the unrefined state because, particularly in the case of grains, it is in the skins, husk, and "germ," that practically the whole store of valuable vitamins and minerals is concealed — put there by an all-wise Providence to counteract the acid-producing effect of the starch.

Avoid the common mistake of "compensating" for a sacrifice of meat by increasing the starch intake. Nature will have to eject it; and catarrhal conditions result, such as: tonsillitis, appendicitis, cholecystitis, leucorrhoea, colds, antrum and sinus disease, urinary frequency and pain, pyelitis, and cystitis.

SENSIBLE COMBINATION. Meals should be simple. On the island of Tristan da Cunha, where teeth are perfect and disease is almost unknown, refined foods don't exist, and the greatest simplicity holds.

In general, since proteins digest in an acid medium, and starches in an alkaline, these foods are best kept apart. Much flatulence and acidity are avoided thereby. Digestion is a process whereby solid foods are dissolved for absorption. Insoluble starchy foods are changed by digestion into glucose; and absorbed in this form. The first step in this process takes place in the mouth by the action of ptyalin, a ferment in the saliva. Thorough mastication ensures effective insalivation.. The changes thus begun are carried on in the stomach and intestines; but are interfered with, even inhibited, in the presence of acid.

When protein foods — meat, cheese, milk, egg-white, fish, and nuts — are swallowed, hydrochloric acid is poured out into the stomach from the cells provided there for the purpose. The hydrochloric acid dissolves the envelopes of the protein molecules, so that the peptone in the gastric juice may act on them.

Hence the inadvisability of consuming, at the same meal, quantities of protein and starchy food. Fermentation, with acid and gas production, results. True, Nature sometimes combines protein and starch — *but in due proportion and form*. It is wise to follow her lead.

The major incompatibilities are easily avoidable, because so little protein or starchy food is required; and either combines satisfactorily with vegetable foods. Fresh fruits combine well with milk or with nuts; but apart from this are best used alone.

Minor discrepancies are irrelevant. Don't become cranky. Better feed foolishly than become food-conscious.

KEEP FOUR POINTS IN MIND:

1. *Don't overeat.*
2. *Shun refined foods.*
3. *Live mainly on vegetables and fruits, as many as possible raw.*
4. *Eat simple meals, avoiding obvious major incompatibilities.*

DO NOT, for want of a little control, allow the body to become acid-poisoned or carbon-clogged; response, both physical, mental, and spiritual, to the dynamic Life Force around and within, will be lessened and depressed if we do; and Disease will be one result.

IN CONCLUSION.

Do not resent restriction. The primary object is nourishment. As in the case when indulgence in alcohol and tobacco is discontinued, discipline and self-control will be rewarded with a disappearance of desire for much that formerly attracted; and a new and increasing enjoyment, relish, and satisfaction will be derived from simple unspoiled foods.

It is amazing that, with what we eat necessarily figuring so prominently in any rational consideration of well being, its importance, even its relevance, should be still almost completely ignored, even scorned and derided, in orthodox medical schools.

In recommending the system of using foods outlined in this book, originality is disclaimed. It has been copied from that in use by Nature Cure Practitioners the world over; and has been particularly adopted from the teaching of Mr Stanley Lief, N.D., D.O., D.C.

The method has been completely vindicated by the findings of the International Defensive Diet League of America; and, while it is not claimed that food cannot be used in any other way, and a fair level of health maintained, this way is advised as the best.

An attempt has been made to spare the disciple the task of devising suitable food combinations by arranging meals in a section on diet in a manner that gets over the difficulty for him.

No effort has been made to treat the subject exhaustively; the scope of this book is indicated in its title. [When "hints" was in the original title.]

ONE FINAL WORD.
God's purpose is to evolve spiritual beings, not animals; and the foods He recommends were contrived to that end.

II. FAULTY GENERAL HABITS
(To be overcome by RIGHT HABITS.)

Brilliant, radiant health may be ours. But it must be earned. It is not for the indolent or self-indulgent. An uncompromising and vital affirmation of the supremacy of the spiritual man will express in discipline and training of the physical vehicle, that it may the more perfectly serve our purpose. A little time must be devoted daily to the care of the body. As it is brought nearer perfection, take a pride in its physical poise and sweet functioning. No longer can there be tolerated the grotesque and flabby caricatures of the glorious instrument God designed to be the temple of His Spirit.

That some old reprobate survives defiance for ninety years is unsound contrary argument. Man should be *living*, today, not merely existing, for a hundred and fifty years. It simply means that some have inherited, usually from frugal-living progenitors, such exceptional constitutions that many years of abuse are needed to break them down. Their children will not prove so lucky.

So many misuse their health to create disease; and not a few, at present quite well, might be better citizens, sick! Life is mental before it is physical; and spiritual before it is either. Let us keep the objective in view!

1. EXERCISE.

Regular exercise is essential. Those who follow a sedentary calling, and all whose life is not an active one, will benefit by daily exercises. A few minutes suffice. The ideal is to exercise, lightly clad, or as nude as conditions permit, in the open. When this is impossible, or inconvenient, exercise naked in the bedroom by an open window. Bending and stretching exercises, with deep breathing, are most health-giving. SELF-MASSAGE, all over, with the bare hands promotes skin activity and healthy function.

A hard walk should be taken every day by all who are prevented from playing games.

After the exercises, have a cold sponge down, dip, or shower; followed by brisk and thorough towelling.

Too little exertion, too much food, choked excretory apparatus, symptoms, wrong treatment, still less exertion, more and worse food, more treatment, eclipse ... and, who will be next!

2. REST.

Sufficient rest is a necessity; but the popular idea of what is required is generally wrong. Not a few people worry over the loss of a few hour's sleep. But it is the worry that hurts, not loss of sleep. Relax quietly and happily, and leave it to Nature. Here as much as anywhere is Right Thinking a necessity. If you cannot sleep, use the time thankfully for fellowship with God.

LEARN TO RELAX. Many sorts of malfunctioning are directly due to a chronic mental bad habit of tension. Rest and smile! During acute elimination, and for recuperative purposes, rest is beneficial. Learn to manifest patience and self-possession.

3. SUN-BATHING.

The exposure of the skin to the sun's rays is one of the essentials of perfect health. If you are not used to it, begin with 5 minutes, about 8 a.m. in the summer, later in winter. Increase by 2 minutes a day up to half an hour. Do NOT sun-bathe in the heat of the day; it is the ultra-violet light rays that do good; the strong heat rays are harmful, and in excessive doses even dangerous.

When conditions do not permit of sun-bathing, have an air-bath quite naked in the bedroom. The skin should be lightly tanned all over, and of a satiny sheen. Grey days are good. SUNLIGHT IS ONE OF THE GREATEST OF ALL THE NATURAL PREVENTIVE AND CURATIVE AGENTS. To deprive children of the protection and invigoration it affords amounts almost to a crime. Let them from their earliest days experience and learn to revel in the daily caress of God's sunshine and air.

4. FRESH AIR.

Life should be lived as far as possible in the open. Avoid congested areas. Never know the smell of stale air. Let buildings and clothing be designed to permit the freest possible circulation of sweet air. The disgusting and foetid atmosphere of thousands of living and sleeping apartments is of itself sufficient to give rise to anaemic, rickety, and scrofulous conditions. In consumptive, asthmatic, and catarrhal conditions generally, the thorough continuous aeration of the breathing passages is one of the fundamental essentials both of prevention and cure. FLAT NARROW CHESTS OF POOR CAPACITY MUST BE DEVELOPED. Stick to it cheerfully and with determination. It is often marvellous what can be achieved with perseverance.

5. *DEEP BREATHING.*

Make a habit of this. Learn to develop and increase chest capacity. Draw deep into the lungs, and so into the blood and whole system, the sweet air and golden sunshine. Greater air-intake means better oxygenation and increased elimination. There are few cases of Asthma (or any other respiratory disorder) that could not have been prevented or cannot completely recover by Right Thinking, Right Food, and methodical TRAINING. I have seen too many recover by perseverance in these simple methods to be deceived as to their efficacy. FAITH, in the outcome; and perseverance!

6. *WATER.*

Within and without. It is the solvent of many of our foods, as of poisonous waste. It bathes and enters into the composition of every living tissue. Drink at least three pints daily; always between meals, never at meals. Water is necessary for cleanliness, to remove the large quantities of dirt excreted through the skin. It is the natural diuretic and diaphoretic. It is a valuable medium for applying heat or cold; and in skilled hands can achieve miracles; as packs and compresses for the relief of pain and localisation and promotion of elimination. As steam it may be inhaled. Diluted with lemon juice it is a valuable antiseptic and dressing for wounds and cavities. To promote elimination, wash the stomach, or encourage bowel activity, drink large quantities.

7. *CLOTHING.*

Should at all times, not forgetting night, be as light and airy as possible. The skin is, or should be, our natural protector from variations in temperature. Unwise and uninstructed parents early rob their children of this valuable function by over-clothing. In adults—that is of course "civilised" adults—this is an almost universal error. Let clothing be spare, but beautiful in colour, texture and design. Colour has a pronounced effect upon mental reaction; and is worthy of study.

8. *POSTURE.*

It is impossible to conceal tone and poise of body (or mind). Posture expresses them. The light and springy step and perfect balance of harmonious vibration; and frank and open gaze; well-cut features, bronzed, and confident with the joy of life; rhythm and grace in movement; as much can be expressed, or betrayed, by posture as by voice. Adopt the posture of assurance, even (or specially!) if at the moment you don't feel it: chin up, shoulders back, chest out, "tummy" in, back straight. This provides the abdominal organs with their natural support. NEVER be persuaded to wear a harness/brace. Sit and stand, TALL, mentally and spiritually as well as physically.

9. *FASTING.*

An occasional short fast is an invaluable prophylactic. Even though we live intelligently, poisons of one kind or another are apt to collect; and it is wise to abstain from food, once in a while, to set the eliminating system free to deal with accumulations. A fast of from three to six days every three months is advised; with a larger one of a week once every year. During these fasts citrus fruit juices, well diluted, and vegetable water should be taken for their eliminative effects; and a daily large enema of two quarts of warm saline should also be used while fasting.

Not only is the physical system cleansed and rejuvenated by this means, but the necessary self-discipline is a valuable moral exercise.

If motive be high enough, what might otherwise be a tiresome penance can become a fascinating pastime: doing our share towards the physical regeneration that will mean new life; and learning the valuable lesson of overcoming sloth, and insincerity of purpose. Many expect "prayer" to restore them to health. It won't. Unless they do their part. We have it within our power to live gloriously, magnificently. Who is willing to manifest his vision!

III. SUPPLY DEFICIENCIES AND PROMOTE ELIMINATION

Merely changing from a wrong way of living to a better one, automatically stimulates elimination. *Vitamin and mineral deficiency and multifarious auto-intoxication* are the great Physical Causes of Disease. Under a more rational regime both these causes are remedied; and the balance, formerly in favour of toxic accumulation, is swung in the other direction. *Vitamin and Mineral Deficiency* may be made good, ideally, by utilizing the alkaline mineral foods. But in systems badly depleted, or with products grown in the usual impoverished soil, extra supplies must be tapped. Preparations of wheat husk and germ, seaweed powdered and dried, extracts of cod—or halibut-liver oil, herbs, and the Homeopathic potentised Cell-salts, all play a part.

To ensure effective supplies while fasting, or if for any good reason whole fruits and vegetables are ineligible, give juices mechanically extracted, or vacuum-packed.

PROMOTING ELIMINATION.

Nothing but experience is likely to carry conviction as to the vast quantities of effete matter often stored in sick bodies. Masses of it, deposited in all sorts of sites in an endeavour to protect vital centres and organs, can be both seen, felt, *and smelt!*

Good health obviously cannot exist with tissues soaked and submerged in this foetid tide. Only Nature (God, that is, the Directive Intelligence within) can remove such encumbrance, and then only through the excretory and eliminative channels provided.

In this, Nature will generally succeed, given a reasonable opportunity and suitable materials.

Manipulative treatment, as every Osteopath and many masseurs are aware, is one of the most useful helps for loosening and mobilizing old stores of sludge. Chiropractic has often indirectly a similar tendency. Neither in hospital nor in private practice can great success be expected where such resources are overlooked.

Hydrotherapy is another of the agencies, familiar to Naturopaths, that work seeming miracles. Hot and cold baths, hot and cold packs, enemas, irrigations, douches, and sprays, all play their part. Combined with instructed manual aid, wonders are often performed. Suitable equipment must be part of the armamentarium of any healing establishment conceived on adequate lines.

Herbs, skilfully chosen and prepared, are often of the greatest possible service, for promoting both re-mineralisation and elimination. This is another branch of the healing art despised and scoffed at by know-alls who never cure. In innumerable instances, even the gravest swellings and growths have been completely dispersed by appropriate herbs, specially when combined with simple general methods.

The Internal Bath. It would be surprising indeed if bodies befouled by filth were not benefited by internal bathing. Those who have not seen the results of washing internally, by drinking large quantities of water, and *working* it through, or of daily rectal injection of quantities as large as five quarts, can have no conception of the condition of many disease-ridden bodies; nor of the regeneration which follows detoxication.

Repeatedly, in medical practice, sick systems soaked beyond saturation point are still further burdened with unusable food and paralysing drugs, while skin eruptions, sewer-like breath, and eliminating systems, generally, in distress, shout aloud what is needed.

The daily enema, when intoxication by retained waste is the cause of the trouble, is perhaps the most effective of all the physical drugless methods of treatment.

Electrical apparatus of many kinds are often of use, as Short wave appliances, Infra-red and Ultra-violet lamps, Diathermy, X-rays, Vibrators, etc.

Dietetic variations, from fasting to full feeding, help powerfully. Make sure, before resorting to eliminative measures, that toxic accumulation is really a factor!

Case-hardened indifference to common-sense feeding comes down heavily on the side of the acid-producers. This trend must be changed by decreasing or even temporarily deleting these foods, and relying largely or solely for a time upon the alkaline elements. *Milk* is one of the main standbys. Thin toxic people, and sufferers from advanced digestive disorder, frequently benefit from quite prolonged periods on a dietary mainly or solely composed of milk. With others, milk forms a basis, with vegetables and fruits in addition. Examples of Eliminating Dietaries are appended later.

Individuals many stones overweight, mineral deficient, and saturated with corruption, must exercise care. Very severe reactions may supervene; and possible danger from this source can be avoided by:

(1) prolonged fasting in suitable cases;

(2) gradual reform, avoiding too sudden a change;

(3) reverting to wrong feeding for a time to check the reactions.

Do not fall into the error of looking upon Nature's way as a method of *treatment*; it is not; it is a manner of living. It is a life-sentence. Backsliding exacts appropriate penalties. Criminals cannot live less a-socially for a few weeks, then return to their crime, and expect to be looked on as cured!

IV. CORRECTING SECONDARY CAUSES

MECHANICAL.

A complete therapeutic system will not ignore the effect upon bodily function of dislocations or subluxations of vertebrae; whether accidental or resulting from toxic conditions.

Many sick individuals — and some well ones too — are benefited by expert Chiropractic and Osteopathic adjustments. In numbers of instances, symptoms can be dispatched by no other means. In others, improvement ensues. Stimulation or inhibition of excretory and secretory action is easily possible. Pain is relieved.

Deformities and disabilities of many kinds are put right by these means. Only the hidebound bigotry of orthodoxy prevents their wider adoption.

Manipulative measures of all kinds, including skilled massage, particularly by responsives who understand something of the operation, through physical contact, of spiritual healing Power, are among the most effective of physical helps.

Discriminating co-relation of all good methods is desirable; for which is worst—trying to reduce displacements by psychological means, or neck-thumping selfish neurotics?

ECONOMIC.

This is among the worst of the secondary causes. Perhaps more than ever today the people languish and anguish and die, for want of a little obedience. Self-interest and financial considerations impede, but need not In an age of unprecedented plenty, any struggle for a living should be an anachronism. Good health and prosperity may be ours almost for the mere taking. Natural resource is unlimited. Productive capacity is virtually as great. We are richer than Croesus. The principal reason we cannot enjoy as much as we like, as well as all that we need, is WE SCRAP FOR IT INSTEAD OF WHACKING IT UP—

> "but if ye bite and devour one another, take heed that ye be not consumed one of another."
>
> Galatians V, 15.

Natural animal man is selfish, greedy, lustful of power, lazy, thriftless, improvident, stupid, ignorant, apathetic. But the greediest, most ruthless and powerful have usurped control of financial wealth.

Such of our real wealth as they permit us access to is capitalised, and the costless corresponding financial "wealth" issued in the form of interest-bearing debt which continually grows.

When, *but never before*, sufficient of us are willing to compete for the common good instead of for gain, we can resume effective control of our credit and currency; and, deciding our policy ourselves, vest responsibility for administration in a body appointed for the purpose.

Instead of heart-breaking taxation we should be drawing dividends from the national increment of association. Emancipation and freedom are within our reach. We must strike off the shackles of moral and financial servitude, and enter into our glorious inheritance as sons and daughters of God.

Balking the banditti, however, will not, alone, solve many problems. So many other factors are involved. Malnutrition, for example, is as much a matter of unwise as of under-indulgence; and self-control is a virtue of Spirit.

8. Helping Nature Cure

I. THE HEALING CRISES

THERE has never been a time when it was more imperative to distinguish between Acute Illness and Disease; because the one is so frequently curative of the other. There is no such thing as Acute Disease. There is Acute Illness; but therein is a vital distinction.

Disease, whether of body, mind, soul, or estate, whether in the individual or the mass, is mostly a gradual degenerative process going on within, due to failure to comply with the requirements of well-being; and, of this process, Acute Illness is commonly Nature's (God's) method of cure.

If Acute Illness is to be understood, the dual significance of symptoms must always be borne in mind. Acute illnesses are not diseases. They are Nature's reactions, curative in intent, against existing disease. They are house cleanings—Healing Crises. Their purpose is warning, disciplinary, protective, eliminative. Through their agency, the body seeks to rid itself of the toxic accumulations which, together with vitamin and mineral deficiency, are the great physical cause of the degenerative process which is disease. Acute Illnesses give sick people a chance to get well. Individuals, people, nation, or world, with integrity threatened by disease, are by such means cleansed, and offered an opportunity of co-operating subsequently in reconstruction.

Acute Illnesses are not primarily dependent upon outside agencies, though they may be precipitated by them. Acute Illnesses commonly arise spontaneously. They should be welcomed and co-operated with, not feared. Acute Illnesses are often man's greatest friend; indeed, had it not been for the Acute Illness, mankind would have ceased to exist long ages ago.

Yet the one really impressive achievement of modern medical "science" consists in suppressing Acute Illnesses! And this, usually, by means shatteringly destructive in themselves.

Orthodox medical men have not the remotest idea as to what these reactions portend. They have been taught to believe that Acute Illnesses are Diseases; that there are hundreds of different ones, each having a specific causative organism; that Nature's glorious redemptive efforts on our behalf are the work of malevolent germs, and must be rigorously repressed at all costs.

Such colossal stupidity is bad enough; but the stubborn refusal to admit what is readily apparent to the average child of tender years, can hardly be too sternly pilloried.

It is galling to watch interminable processions of people plainly loaded, bloated, and blocked with debris derived from ignorance, indulgence, and gluttony, being prodded and tapped and thumped, tested and listened to, X-Rayed, and investigated, observed and consulted about, then butchered, or poisoned, or burned; while in Toxic Accumulation, their symptoms have one common origin which Nature will often correct if given a chance.

Being content to earn a living from treating symptoms, and leaving their causes unchallenged and still active, either in the individual or the mass, will soon be labelled dishonest. To keep the mind closed to new truth for fear of possible consequences, economic or otherwise, betrays lack of faith; but may be just as dishonest.

THE GOSPEL OF "NATURE CURE."

There is little to fear from disease, for those content to live healthily. If people were half as afraid of living unhealthily as they are today of disease, there would be little left of disease.

People are sometimes disturbed and confounded when, at more or less regular intervals after adopting a healthier regime, disturbances still crop up; but, having set yourself to live better, when Nature reacts, either in body, mind, soul, or estate, don't be perturbed! It is a grand and radiant message—the Gospel of Good!

If symptomatic warnings of the presence of disease have been ignored, and measures for dealing with the causes neglected, sooner or later, even though the causes continue, Nature will stage a reaction. The road back to health is frequently punctuated by temporary apparent set-backs, in the form of more or less mild Acute Illnesses; and it is essential to understand their significance, and to know what to do when they occur.

THESE ARE NATURE'S HEALING CRISES.

Yet, so ingrained is the fear of disease as evil attacking from without that, despite reiterated and most painstaking instruction, the significance of these sudden disturbances is still constantly overlooked, and the customary suppressive measures resorted to.

Often enough, in those grossly burdened with poisons of many varieties, a Healing Crisis may be a formidable experience. But the folly of foiling such purpose by trying to force in food, and paralysing the life-saving cleansing apparatus with vaccines or drugs, must surely be evident. Have nothing to do with such.

Beware of orthodox methods, which, being so frequently wrong in principle, can hardly be expected to work satisfactorily in practice.

When we've got over our fear of Acute Illness, we shall have broken the back of the disease bogey; so drop that insensate fear of disease. Practise confidence. God and Nature are on our side, even if modern medicine is mostly opposed. The body is a self-cleansing "machine," and running to a medical man, after years of indulgence and wrong thinking to have the healing crises suppressed, is little better than suicide.

NATURE'S EFFORTS TO CURE. THEIR ONSET, AND ACTION.

HEALING CRISES usually develop quite unexpectedly to those who don't understand; often after a spell of most gratifying improvement. They are usually ushered in either by gradually developing "seediness," or more suddenly by shivering, rise of temperature, loss of appetite, furred tongue, rapid breathing and pulse, burning skin, assorted aches and pains, headache, and general malaise.

According to the kind and quantity of poisons, and eliminating organs chosen, appearances vary when reaction sets in. Exaggeration or recurrence of old familiar symptoms is to be expected at such times. The taste of drugs taken or injected long years before may even be identified.

Particular symptoms, such as catarrhal elimination, sore throat, diarrhoea, biliousness, rashes, or cough may appear, according to the channel or channels selected by the inner Directive Intelligence.

Generally, all channels are in action. Fever, caused by fermentation of stored-up waste, is Nature's bonfire. The tongue becomes coated, signifying the condition of inner surfaces and linings, which, like the outer skin, are being used for elimination. The breath becomes foul, because an assortment of putrid material is being thrown out through the lungs and linings of the breathing passages and apparatus. Sputum is sometimes copious, when mucous filth is extruded. Antra and sinuses may become choked for a time. Skin eruptions, boils, rashes, and carbuncles may appear; or deeper seated abscesses, when waste is concentrated in organs, cavities, or connective-tissue planes. Volumes of foetid filth are sometimes thrown out through the liver, or lining of stomach, and vomited up. Diarrhoea is the usual mode of ejecting irritant substances excreted through intestinal glands or mucosa. The urinary tract may exhibit signs of disturbance: pain, aching, frequency, burning, urgency, inflammation, in kidneys, ureters, bladder, or urethra. The urine is likely to be loaded with solid matter in solution or suspension; and, if the poisons are highly toxic in character, there may be temporary damage to tissue. Purulent or mucous discharge from the vagina is common, with accompanying symptoms of deeper discomfort.

Such are the evidences that Nature is now prepared to throw out, in bulk, poisons which hitherto she had been trying to eliminate piecemeal.

Diphtheria, measles, boils, carbuncles, abscesses, bronchitis, pneumonia, scarlet fever, tonsillitis, quinsy, antrum, sinus and mastoid "infection," pyelitis, nephritis, cystitis, colds, salpingitis, are neither Diseases, nor Diagnoses, they are merely the *names* of everyday examples of Healing Crises.

DURATION.

The duration of a Healing Crisis is dependent upon a number of factors; for instance: — the amount and toxicity of collected-up poisons; the degree of bodily strength and vitality; the effectiveness or otherwise of measures adopted; the mental reaction of patient, relatives, and "friends"; the extent of previous orthodox "treatment." Generally, a reaction will last from one to three or four days; but may extend to ten or twelve days; exceptionally, much longer.

When the system has been badly poisoned for years, and specially where orthodox suppressive or "preventive" treatment has been carried out, a considerable period of time is likely to elapse, punctuated by a succession of healing efforts, before regeneration and reconstruction can become well advanced. *It may easily be many years before the process can be complete.* Improvement may quite well continue indefinitely, in those who loyally persevere. Nature's methods are deliberate; too much so, often, for impatient humanity (which is one reason for the popularity still enjoyed by those who presume to offer a quick but illusory alternative).

THE PERIODICITY OF DISEASE.

After a period of mistaken living, or, in the case of infants, at varying but often surprisingly regular intervals after their arrival in the world heavily charged with hereditary and maternal toxins, *Nature will stage a reaction.* Many of the disorders of early life are explained in this way.

As in most other human concerns, critical periods recur, in health and disease, in major and minor cycles of six and seven – days, weeks, months, years, decades, centuries, and millennia.

FIVE, in spiritual numerics, is the figure of flux. SIX is directional. SEVEN is fruitional; and indicative of Spiritual plan, process, and purpose.

No very extensive experience is needed in Natural Methods of healing before attention is arrested by the almost uncanny recurrence of these significant numbers.

Very frequently, but by no means invariably, Healing Crises occur in the 6th, 13th, or 20th weeks, or in the 6th, 13th, or 20th months, from the commencement of an improved regime, or course of corrective treatment. Further reactions may appear in the 6th, 13th, or 20th years.

PARENTHETICALLY.

It is relevant to note that the world is now at the dawning of the millennium—a circumstance directly connected with the present World Epoch of cosmic accelerating intensity. This epoch is moving daily nearer a Crisis. A grand-scale Reaction impends —a mass clean-up, with heavy mortality and discharge of diseased and spiritually dead individuals, or "cells."

As with bodies sick unto death, the Adamic "patient" will be brought desperately low in the process—to the very verge of extinction. It will appear for a time like the end of all law and order: the triumph of anarchy. *It is the fluxing of the old evil order, preparatory to the inmoving of the new.*

PROCEDURE.

Except in the gravely debilitated, whenever a Healing Crisis supervenes, of more than evanescent proportions, A FAST SHOULD BE UNDERTAKEN IMMEDIATELY, and all relevant measures adopted to facilitate elimination. NO FOOD WHATEVER should be given in most cases, not even milk.

If food is given, elimination may be interfered with, and Nature's beneficent purpose delayed and even prevented. It is for this reason that so many acute symptoms are allowed to become chronic; and so many lives lost which might easily have been saved.

Let no one listen to those who would urge food "for strength to fight the germs (or the disease)"; it is the germs that will use the food, and the patient will suffer.

II. THE PART PLAYED BY FASTING

The body may be likened, roughly, to a sponge, which can either absorb, or squeeze out; but cannot reasonably be expected to do both, efficiently, at one and the same time. Remember the animals — they know what to do. But animals follow their instinct; while man's instinct is betrayed by misaligned reason, which deludes him into the belief that Nature's Healing Crises are the work of truculent microbes.

Precipitating causes must be distinguished from primary. Do not be misled, even if acute illness has been precipitated by some external influence. "Chills" do not ordinarily make healthy people diseased, neither do germs.

If Nature, by the sudden onset of illness, signalises her intention of undertaking active remedial measures, it will be the part of wisdom to do all in our power to further her purpose. And bear in mind that Nature cannot be expected to alter her laws to suit our convenience.

FASTING, in the management of disease, should be limited in the main to two kinds of disorder:

1. Fasting, usually partial but sometimes complete, will be necessary in most cases of Acute Illness.
2. Fasting is a rapid promoter of detoxication in those, otherwise sufficiently robust, whose symptoms are predominantly *Toxic*.

CAUTION.

Deficiency and accumulation are constantly present together. Where deficiency preponderates, fasting must be conducted discreetly; otherwise existing shortage may be increased, and weakness made worse. Also, in subjects profoundly poisoned, with vitality greatly depressed, the severity of toxaemia evoked and of healing reactions provoked, might prove too great. Remember the purpose of fasting—to facilitate elimination. Fasting is not a "cure." Do not permit the feeble, debilitated, asthenic, or consumptive to fast—except under *expert* direction.

Fasting should be carried out, always, under supervision of one who understands the procedure. Like the knife, in skilled hands, fasting is capable of wonderful good; but unskilfully employed becomes a dangerous weapon. Nicest discrimination is needed.

Nearly all acute, and many chronic symptoms, yield to fasting; but to attempt to elaborate directions to cover all types of case would be to venture far beyond the scope of this book.

Children of parents whose MENTAL OUTLOOK IS RIGHT, who are fed correctly and obey the other rules of right living, will seldom be troubled by disease; but if symptoms appear do not be afraid. *Confidence* is your life-line: don't relinquish your hold when you encounter rapids. That's when we need it most. Put the child to bed, use the enema at once and repeat it each day, begin a fast, apply hot and cold packs alternately to the seat of pain or disturbance, give copious drinks—not milk, of course, which is a food—stimulate skin activity, and parents will be gratified by the rapid disappearance of the trouble.

DURATION OF A FAST.

In acute illness, the fast must, generally, be continued until the symptoms have completely subsided. This is not invariably the case, because the patient's strength may not be equal to the strain. It may sometimes be necessary to break the fast, and wait for a subsequent reaction to complete the clean up. There is nothing to fear; on the contrary, there is every reason for thankfulness that God, through His natural law, has provided such effective protection from the consequences of wilfulness and stupidity.

The longest fasts personally supervised are, in a child of 10 months, 14 days; in a child of 18 months, 19 days; in a man of 67 years, 63 days. Three other people have fasted over 40 days, and two or more between 30 and 40 days. Fasts of over 20 days even are rare. The usual duration of a fast, either in acute or chronic disorder, is from one or a few, to (occasionally) fourteen days.

Where the system is soaked in accumulated toxins, and Nature has set herself to get rid of them, it will be foolish to break the fast, unless the patient's condition demands it. Do not allow ignorance and fear to deprive the patient of his chances of recovery.

In the chronic manifestations, we must be guided by circumstance. If symptoms are still present, the breath foul, the tongue heavily coated, enema returns still dirty, urine thick on standing, and strength reasonably well maintained, it will generally be wise to continue.

Naturally, weight will be lost; but as those whose systems are badly poisoned are, as a rule much overweight, this is all to the good.

In any case, if we have got ourselves into such a condition, we must be prepared to make some contribution towards reprieve.

Large numbers of people have fasted ninety to one hundred days on water alone. But don't fast foolishly; and do not act at all unless Nature's regenerative purpose is served.

A man, 67 years of age, told by the doctors, and "specialists," in two different towns, that "nothing could be done for him," fasted 63 days on orange juice, water, and vegetable water. The fast was undertaken when, at the end of three weeks on the Standard Diet, a reaction appeared in the form of "tonsillitis," temperature, assorted rheumatic pains, and general malaise. When treatment began he could not even stand without crutches; and could manage only a very short distance with their help. This condition, of rheumatism and thrombosis, had been developing for years; much more rapidly during the last 12 months. After 30 days' fast, the patient was walking a mile every day. After 6 weeks' fast, he was walking 4 miles every day. After 8 weeks' fast, he was walking 6 miles every day. On the 63rd day of his fast, he walked 10 miles; and having completed the distance, smilingly protested his obvious ability to repeat the performance. It was estimated that the quantity of poisonous filth eliminated through the bowel alone was in the neighbourhood of two benzine tins full. The fast was now gradually broken; the formerly hopeless invalid swinging along, the while, with a stride four feet long and grinning from ear to ear.

Ten months later he wrote:

> There can't be much wrong with the treatment, for I walked 16 miles on Friday, 12 miles on Saturday, took

three services in widely scattered localities on Sunday, walking the whole distance; had a warm bath, and feel as fit as I did 30 years ago and am still steadily improving!

Where disease is of very long standing, do not expect miracles. These happen only under special circumstances, which perhaps is as well. Blessings cheaply obtained are too cheaply valued. Likewise, systems hereditarily sickly, and undermined by long years of misdeeds, cannot be rejuvenated by five minutes' repentance. But do your best— repentance may be deferred, but can't be evaded;

"except ye repent, ye shall all likewise perish"

Jesus Christ.

PHENOMENA COMMONLY OBSERVED DURING A FAST.

If a mud bottomed pool is stirred with a stick, dirt will come to the top. Fasting is such a stick. In the effort to safeguard our health, Nature will deposit all waste which she cannot eliminate, as far as possible in non-vital localities. In grossly toxic systems, poison will be deposited in intercellular spaces and intermuscular planes; in connective tissue and fascial structures; in tendon sheaths and lymphatic system; while every cell will contain its quota. Toxic accumulation in any particular organ, complicated by bacterial action, may have destructive effect; but the damage will generally be repaired when the offending toxins have gone.

During a fast, in the initial stage of increased toxaemia, there is often a feeling of weakness, dizziness, or goneness at the knees; but this is transitory, and after four or five days, is succeeded by a sensation of relief, and an access of energy, that gives assurance of improvement.

Contrary to natural expectation hunger is seldom a feature. If such is in evidence, it is almost certainly due to entertaining longings or thoughts about food. "Habit hunger" may have to be controlled for a day or two; but does not, as a rule, present any real difficulty.

In general, when Nature has achieved her purpose, the discharge of offensive matter from the bowel will cease; the tongue will gradually clear; and natural hunger return. This is a signal to begin breaking the fast. Where there are massive accumulations of drugs and general waste, no fast, however prolonged, is likely to cleanse the system completely. The clearing of the tongue is only one indication; and fasts are often broken with the tongue still furred.

The Lord Jesus fasted 40 days; not as a meaningless gesture, but for the purpose of cleansing His system to increase sensitivity, receptivity, and response. And "was afterward anhungered." Like any one else on a fast, hunger was not in evidence till His system was clean.

9. Mental And Spiritual Healing

"Now faith is the assurance of things hoped for, the proving of things not seen."

Hebrews XI, 1. (RV.)

I. FAITH HEALING

THE natural regenerative process set in operation by all the foregoing can be intensified and accelerated, potentially to any degree, through FAITH. And faith, in its simplest sense, is the child-like certainty that the Divine Healing POWER, though invisible, is present, adequate, and at work.

Faith is quiet rejoicing assurance of well-being *already existing*; it is also confidence, courage, cheerfulness, determination, and perseverance; which are faith in action.

Do not mistake, for faith, acquiescence in religious dogma, or profession of belief in a distant but more than half .dreaded deity. The professing are, too often, bigoted, intolerant, uncontrolled; and, not infrequently, less responsive than the average. Belief alone is inadequate. Belief is the starting point; but faith is the venture whereby belief is transformed into experience. And experience begets understanding; and understanding, spiritual consciousness.

Faith is the faculty that makes contact with the impalpable; that clothes with reality that of which the senses bear no witness.

Faith is the switch that sets in operation the potentially unlimited spiritual Life-Force inherent within. The size of the switch is irrelevant. It is the position that counts — on or off. Faith the size of a mustard seed will remove mountains — if backed up by "works."

Faith is operative to the degree of spiritual sensitivity, receptivity, and response. The law, *in relativity*, is "According to your faith be it unto you." That is, in measure, according to the direction of faith, negative or positive, it will be unto us—evil or good. Pious protestation cannot counter-balance the effects of negative faith.

The physically-conscious need props for their faith. Faith in medicine, faith in a doctor, faith in a procedure, faith in a chiropractic manoeuvre, faith in a "diet," faith in a piece of the true cross (which may have come from somebody's barn door), faith in one's ability to recover, faith in anything; it matters little *so long as the subconscious mind is sufficiently impressed with the recovery concept*. But the most powerful and effective incentive to faith must be a consciousness of the nature and source of the Healing Power within.

Most people swallow their food in faith. They know little or nothing of how it works; but it reappears in due course as energy, heat, and waste. So also with the mind. We should not forbear to accept the power of Spirit to heal because we do not fully or at all understand how He works. Accept the assurance in faith, and in like course it will materialise as healing or other desired objective.

Not faith in some outside "god" is required; but faith in recovery, faith to persist, faith in essential goodness and life; faith that all is well, particularly when most apparently or obviously ill. How many manage quite nicely till faith meets some test, in danger or difficulty? Then physical consciousness lets go the lifebelt, and, striking out on its own, is quickly engulfed.

Everybody adopts one of two alternatives. Either we allow untoward outward appearances to work back through our minds and impress or depress our true spiritual selves; or, realising our spiritual nature and continuity with limitless Power, we set that Power to work, by faith, outwardly through our minds to bring back into harmony whatever in physical selves or circumstances was seeming discordant.

Never let outward appearances impress, *no matter how menacing. Know one thing only — His presence, His nature, His instant accessibility, and His absolute unchallengeable Power.*

The Faith that heals takes no account of appearances, however imposing. Faith does not reason. Faith KNOWS. The spiritual creative Power must always be greater than material created things:

"Greater is He that is in You, than he that is in the world."
1 John IV, 4.

Faith must be present in the healer; if possible in the sufferer; and is more than helpful in relatives and friends. Its force is stepped up by intensity of desire to be made *whole*, within and without; by purity of motive; and by clarity of grateful perception. Mighty resources are waiting to honour our faith, but — once again, beware its direction.

It is not merely foolish to worry: it is actively dangerous, and not infrequently fatal. Worry is fear; and "fear is faith in evil"; and according to our faith it will be unto us. Faith is the thought or belief at the back of our inmost mind. To fear disease is to invite and create disease. To fear poverty is to make shortage inevitable. To fear danger or accident is to encounter recurring woe. Fear of failure ensures it. Fear of evil sets in operation the mysterious invisible mind forces that materialise evil. "For the thing which I greatly feared is come unto me," mourned the once greatly-blessed Job, "and that which I was greatly afraid of has come unto me."

To most, the world is disquietingly material: a place of dark foreboding and imminent danger. To clearer perception, life is a state of consciousness in which our conceptions become accurately embodied in circumstances and physical selves.

Mere common sense would urge the advisability of essaying a venture in faith. Either there is, or is not, an omnipotent beneficent Power. We had better decide, and take GOOD for granted—simply act on the assumption that GOOD will come, in body, mind, soul and estate—that is what brings it to pass!

That which distinguishes human beings, "alive," from their physical bodies, "dead," is the presence, within, of Life Energy. That Life Energy or Life Force, is Spirit. Theologians call that Life Spirit—"GOD"; and we, are part of, and continuous with, not separate from, Eternal, Indestructible, Spirit. We are individualisations of that "GOD," or Spirit of GOOD. He is not merely powerful without limit—"the Power that swings the suns": He is also boundlessly wise and intelligent—the Power that contrived and controls our intricate body chemistry. He is also absolutely benevolent (Christ showed us that); infinitely patient, and perfectly loving: longing to take control. And faith (AND *obedience*) afford Him the sanction He needs. *Ponder* this therefore: we, and that Spirit, are ONE.

St Paul, the greatest healer, save One, of whom we have record, who showed by results that he knew what he did, advised "Be ye transformed by the renewing of your minds."

Paraphrasing for the sake of clearness, Hebrew idiom and old English translation might better be rendered thus "If you want to be transformed, *change your mental outlook*"—that is, from sickness to health, from poverty to abundance, from doubt and misgiving to confidence and certainty, from selfishness to eager self-forgetfulness, from weakness to strength, from hate to love, from fear to glad faith, from negative to positive, from evil to GOOD, in fact from physical to spiritual.

"CAN GOD?"

For twenty-five years "Lofty" had been a criminal. Fifteen years of that time he had spent in gaol. Coming out for the last time, his evil nature aflame, he swore to avenge himself; and began to drink.

Slouching along the dark streets late one evening, after ten days on cheap liquor and methylated spirits, he stumbled unawares into a little "mission for down and outs."

There, through the efforts of three sincere-minded men, Lofty, soaked to the tips of his dirty hair with vile booze, experienced "conversion"—was induced, that is, to change his mental outlook and habit of mind.

Sickened beyond endurance by his pitiable plight, and by sufferings self-inflicted through long years of vicious indulgence, his stubborn resistance was humbled at last. The Spirit within, fortified through the mediation of others, was able to change his direction; and the regenerative process began. Lofty co-operated willingly and wholeheartedly.

Months later, still financially down and out and a martyr to indigestion, he was given a battered old lorry. Later, he traded this for a better one; and, later again, secured a brand new machine. In less than three years he owned a fine fleet of four vehicles.

Shown the cause of digestive disorder, he had his teeth put to rights, and began to use foods more wisely. His digestion completely recovered. That happened seven years ago, and today, even without opening his mouth, Lofty preaches a challenging sermon; for everyone knows what he was, and even a fool can see what he is.

Through repentance, faith, and obedience, the degenerative process was arrested and converted into a regenerative process. This will continue "till he comes in the unity of the faith, and of the knowledge of the son of God, unto a perfect man, unto the measure of the stature of the fullness of Christ."

II. HOW FAITH WORKS

Faith asks, and receives, and believes it has; spiritual conscious knows IT IS.

The justification for faith is that man is a spiritual being, part of and continuous with, not separate from, the Divine Creative Living Loving Life Force referred to as GOD. That Force is solely and only and always GOOD. In Spirit, He is what the Lord Jesus showed Him to be; and in His Law He is perfect.

One great stumbling block has been the apparent reality, solidity, and permanence of matter. To material sense things look so very dense and convincing. Yet nothing exists that is not Spirit.

Matter, the physicists tell us, is merely a form of electrical energy; and electrical energy is spiritual energy in lower vibration. Reduced to its ultimate components, matter, whether diamond, wood, water, flesh, bone or blood, is found to consist of atoms; the atoms of molecules; the molecules of positive and negative charges of electricity (and neutrons) revolving round one another as separately as stars in the sky. (Note the polarity!)

Spirit is the source of electrical energy. Mind is the medium through which that energy works. Thought is the instrument that sets it to work, and determines the direction in which it shall work, positive constructive or negative destructive. Matter is the field in which results are produced. Mind is the medium between Spirit and matter; the spoken word is the link.

The different material appearances vary according to the number, arrangement, and rate of vibration of the electrical charges composing them. These variations are mind controlled. Matter is Spirit reduced in vibratory frequency to a point where it becomes sense-perceptible: which frequency is infinitely variable. Matter is Spirit in relativity—is, in fact, very largely, our consciousness, or impression of Spirit.

It is said of Christ, Philippians II, 6, that He was "in the form of God." But God, of course, has no "form." The Greek for "in the form of" is "en morphe," meaning, "the impression made by a person or thing on the vision or senses." Men did not "see" Christ. We do not see, feel, hear, taste, or smell anything; we receive sense impressions of mental conceptions, or misconceptions, of spiritual ideas.

Those who saw the Lord Jesus Christ received a visual (and intuitional) impression of God, Spirit; which is why Jesus said "he that hath seen Me hath seen the Father."

VITAL CONSIDERATIONS.

Man's idea of himself as material, weak, sick, sinful and limited (and his animal failings derive therefrom) is man's mistaken conception due to consciousness underdeveloped. God's idea of man is perfect—"made in His image and likeness."

There is only One Source of healing or health. ALL healing is of the Spirit, and comes from within. Usually, indwelling Spirit will make us well, when we stop making ourselves ill. This Natural healing process, universally operating, is fortified strongly by faith—confidence, that is, in wholeness (the inward reality actually existing) ; and faith is steeply increased by developing consciousness of our continuity with the One Divine Source of ALL GOOD.

Grains of dry sand thinly spread on a sheet of metal arrange themselves, under the vibratory influence of music nearby, in geometrical patterns. If discords be struck, the pattern becomes confused; to be correctly disposed once more when harmony reigns again.

Matter is Spirit, and thought links the two. Negative thought is the discordant note. (Even disease originating in the physical, through ignorant infraction of Law, is made worse, many-fold, by fear and disease consciousness.) With obedience restored and natural healing efforts cooperated with on the physical plane, re-harmonising the determining thought vibrations through confidence in wholeness MUST re-arrange disordered electrical charges.

Thought forces thus re-harmonised are raised in vibratory rate by growing consciousness, through spiritual meditation, uplifting influence of people of higher understanding, and the direct drawing power of Spirit.

Wrong appearances or manifestations, in self or surroundings, must be due to a mistaken impression of things as they really are:

"and God SAW everything that He had made, and, behold, it was very GOOD."

Genesis I, 31.

What is needed is to identify the error, and correct the wrong impression by knowing and so "seeing" the Truth.

The physical-minded hope for improvement *first, before* reversing the destructive thoughts responsible for their miseries. But "the just shall live by faith," not by sight.

Perceiving the self-evident folly of holding between Spirit and matter the kind of thought inevitably materialising sickness and poverty, and realising our identity and heritage as perfect spiritual beings, the greatest service we can render (given repentance, obedience, and co-operation), must be, by clear inner perception, to hold the hesitant on truth's "ultra-violet," fine-vibrational, carrier wave of love, and faith.

Our task, to the degree of sensitivity, receptivity, and response of our "wireless instrument," is to mediate and instruct.

"GREATER THINGS THAN THESE."

Man's materialising mechanism is clumsy and crude in the lower "times"; but as sensitivity evolves and consciousness unfolds he gradually transcends material limitation of any kind. Man makes (and bakes), by the sweat of his brow. But methods evolve, as response to Spirit increases and grasp of the Law improves. Ultimately, stones may be made bread, or two loaves a thousand, as understanding develops.

The Lord Jesus, by the power of thought, could materialise His supply direct from invisible Spirit. He could see or heal at any distance. He could walk on the water; and raise or subdue a storm. He could lower or raise His own vibratory rate at will, and appear or vanish from sight as He pleased. Walls could not contain nor death hold dominion over Him. But whatever He thought or did was always in perfect submission of self to the "Father Within."

But remember the Law, which Christ Himself said He came to fulfil, not to destroy. Spirit has no means of expression, except through the Law. Spirit cannot express successfully in defiance of His own Law—His own safeguards of well-being! The Law is inviolable, and spiritual beings, though no longer in bondage thereto, are still under the Law.

But inexorable as is the Law, *salvation (well-being) cannot come by the Law, which fails owing to the weakness of the flesh.* Right thinking, right feeding; and right acting, while conducive to higher development, do not necessarily ensure it. *Redemption is of the Spirit; and expresses as obedience to the Law.*

POWER UNLIMITED.

Electrical energy, for all practical purposes unlimited, is carried in wires outside our homes. Inside are lamps, radio, heaters, cleaners and cookers; but if we are ignorant of or misapply the laws which govern its use, instead of light, music, comfort, and food, the power may produce fires and shocks.

So too with our bodies; they are actually composed of, not merely surrounded by spiritual electrical Energy, potentially unlimited. But, exactly as with its lower vibratory homologue, unless we learn and obey the laws which govern right functioning, in place of health, happiness, safety and prosperity —poverty, disease, disaster and death will result.

In neither case is the power at fault. The power is impersonal. Evil is mostly man-made; and can only be man unmade, and then only in perfect accord with Infinite Spirit AND Law.

The limitless secrets of immeasurable Wisdom, Knowledge, and Understanding are progressively revealed to responsive, polarised man through spiritual intuition.

THE JUSTIFICATION FOR FAITH.

FEAR is the GREAT cause of disease. Not necessarily fear of anything in particular; just sheer LACK OF CONFIDENCE—settled belief in present or impending mischance.

The one blazing vindication of faith is—IT WORKS! Realising, BY FAITH to begin with, that God is not an individual who lives in the sky, nor yet in some far-away *place*, called Heaven, that God is everywhere present around *and within*, that God IS what Christ showed Him to be, that He can and does, to the degree of our response, actually, from within, order our lives for us with infinite wisdom and absolute dependability, ALL FEAR IS BANISHED FOR EVER.

Never again for the rest of eternity need we have one least fleeting qualm. Henceforth, given willingness and co-operation, HE WILL increasingly LIVE HIS LIFE in our thoughts and actions.

There is no such thing as death. Life cannot be destroyed. Its "form" may be changed. But life is eternal—"the gift of God is eternal life"—and the change we call death is merely the somewhat clumsy procedure whereby we enter the next stage of our endless God-guided unfoldment. Deepening consciousness brings realisation that the "Kingdom of Heaven IS at hand." We may dwell there now, and continue our sojourn to the end of unending time with the Spirit of GOOD and His Christ. Thus the best of our life is still to come; and, what is more, THAT WILL ALWAYS BE TRUE.

"CHRIST IN YOU, THE HOPE OF GLORY."

"In all these things we are more than conquerors through Him Who loved us."

You who are sick! Can you be persuaded, NOW, once and for all to drop EVERY fear and wrong thought—all stubborn clinging to belief in the reality and power of disease; in the ability of the material appearances you have created, to dominate the power that created and is maintaining them?

Disease, crime, poverty, are mostly bad habits of mind. The misery arising therefrom can't be got rid of without giving up their cause. If we want Disease to go out of our bodies, or circumstances, we MUST let the thought of or belief in Disease go out of our minds.

GOD IS REAL. PUT HIM TO THE TEST. ACCEPT His assurance. How *can* we expect to receive that which we do not or *will* not accept? In Spirit (and therefore in *reality*), perfection, health, goodness, prosperity, are our true condition NOW. There is nothing that is not GOD! How may that statement be proved? —By taking GOOD for granted, now, henceforth, and for ever: THAT, TOO, IS FAITH IN ACTION.

A small effort of will is required to take the first step: finally to abandon the mulish wrong habit of mind: to "snap out" of that selfish *practice* of fear, disease, or self-pity. But the reward is commonly so out of all proportion to the smallness of the contribution demanded, that *most are fools to be sick.*

Are you *willing* to be made *whole*? Then PROVE IT, in the only way possible: by ceasing to make yourself ill!

Do you believe? In Whom; or in what? In GOOD; or in ill? *Lord, help thou our unbelief!*

Instead of being everlastingly wrapped up in ourselves, and whining about our hard luck, shall we make up our minds to contribute to the sum total of happiness and love by, continually, giving these out? *That's how we get them in!*

FAITH, REPENTANCE, AND OBEDIENCE. Too high a price? We shall find the cost is only that which was formerly spoiling our life.

So plug in! Switch on! THE POWER IS THERE. But make *certain* that you have truly let go that last scrap of selfishness, doubt, or wrong thought, at the very back of your mind. (If there's the tiniest doubt or misgiving, then, actually, the thought is unchanged.)

STOP FIGHTING. GIVE IN, NOW! "LET GO, AND LET GOD." And trust HIM, utterly and for ever. But see that, henceforth, we walk, with all the zeal we can summon, the way of the Spirit. Climb; even tho' we slip.

SEEK, *FIRST*, the Kingdom of GOOD, and His Right-use-ness; *everything* else (given obedience to the Law) just naturally falls into place.

"Watch ye, stand fast in the faith, quit you like men, BE STRONG."

1 Corinthians XVI, 13.

"WE AND OUR FATHER ARE ONE."

III. HIGHER HEALING RESOURCES

"Behold, I will bring to it health and healing, and I will heal them and reveal to them abundance of prosperity and security."

Jeremiah XXXIII, 6.

ABSENT TREATMENT.

Thought transference is an established fact; and in those of high receptivity exerts a potent effect. It is one of the latent resources.

Dense physical texture, negative bias, gross defilement, enfeebled heredity, reduce response.

Thought transference, being a vibrational force, operates best by contact; hence the laying on of hands. Virtue comes through the healer, not the device. But Spirit knows limitation neither of time nor space; and distance is no bar to His working.

Concentration in higher consciousness upon any in need, however far distant, has produced phenomena too familiar to need reiteration. Because of the unity of Spirit, most spiritual-mental methods profitable when sufferers are present, are equally efficacious, quite frequently more so, at a distance. Given co-operation, results are often most gratifying; even without their knowledge, continually holding an individual in the thought of wholeness and spiritual perfection, giving wholehearted thanks for deliverance, protection, provision, health, already existing, secures their fulfilment. Man cannot receive (or invent), what does not already exist; the only difficulty is in letting *consciousness* dawn, of that which, within, is already complete. Where the necessitous one's vision is holden, we can "see" for him.

Whether through contact or at a distance, perfect realisation of harmony in the Absolute will manifest in its relative expression; and in those sufficiently evolved expresses as miracle.

PRAYER.

Mild surprise is excusable at widespread persistence in supplication for assorted benefits which never materialise. Surface, unthinking pietism, invariably one hundred per cent unproductive, should be hard to defend! But men are not taught to think: they are carefully taught not to think. Not one in a thousand has ever attempted the feat.

Prayer, in the still generally-accepted sense, for the sick, may make them much worse. To hold thoughts of pain and disease about people is sending destructive vibration. Fortunately, those who "pray" thus do not use their mental utensil; and prattling pious good wishes has little effect either way.

Do not pray and pray for a God some look upon, mistakenly, as outside of and separate from ourselves, to relent and reluctantly grant that which, by His Spirit, the Christ within, He is striving His utmost to have us accept.

To a great extent man answers his prayers himself. Prayer is concentration. Prayer is dominant desire, often disguised. But beware the thought or belief deeper down, for, GOOD, BAD, INDIFFERENT, DESIRED, OR FEARED, the idea or impression at the back of our minds will materialise; and not, unless closely identified with it, the more superficial wish many miscall prayer.

TRUE PRAYER IS BRINGING DESIRE INTO CONFORMITY WITH THE DIVINE PURPOSE AND WILL.

"Before they call, I will answer."

Isaiah LXV, 24.

True prayer is receptivity—"picking up," "boosting," and "re-broadcasting," the wireless of the Spiritual Kingdom. Hence the compelling necessity of co-operating to increase sensitivity.

Prayer is a mighty force, perhaps the greatest we have. Rightly understood, it can effect the greatest good; but wrongly applied is capable of almost infinite harm. Any thought strongly and tenaciously held tends to materialise; and, great as is this power, the effect of the spoken word is greater still; sung, it is greatest of all.

For eleven years J. M. had been unemployed and was unemployable on account of "Asthma." The last time he left hospital, the Medical Superintendent said to him: "J., there's always a bed for you if you have to come back; but if the man is living that can ever really do anything for you, I'll agree it's a miracle!"

For weary months this case was laboured upon. Persistently encouraged, in face of almost every conceivable discouragement (much of it deliberate), J. did his best. He gave up poisoning himself with tobacco and alcohol; he subsisted on a tightly restricted diet; he underwent fasts; he exercised, perseveringly; and learned how to breathe. For several months, progress was disappointingly slow. Then he began to improve more quickly.

After a year and a half he was well enough to make a start with some work; and the problem of finding a job presented itself. It was solved by PRAYER — in this way:

His wife, a sincere church goer, was asked: "Mrs. M., why don't you get your husband a job?"

"How do you mean," she queried. "Prayer?"

"Of course!" was the reply.

"But, Doctor," she objected. "I've prayed every night for over twelve years!"

"What! . . . Well, no wonder he's been sick! You can't know much about prayer! . . . What do you *do* when you pray?"

"I kneel down, and ask God to cure J., and find him a job."

"Excellent! But . . . what thought is in your mind while you do that?"

"Why, the thought that I want him well, and in work."

"Yes," was agreed, "that, no doubt, is the thought in the front of your mind. But think a minute—what is the real thought, *right at the very back of your mind?*"

The real thought was not so very far back after all, for almost at once Mrs. M. burst out:

"What would be the thought at the back of my mind, with my husband tortured almost to death, and the children half starved, and the rent owing, and no clothes to our backs. . ."

"That" (very gently), "is exactly the point, Mrs. M.! It isn't what we *say*, with our superficial mind, to something or someone we conceive of, mistakenly, as outside of and separate from ourselves, whom we call 'God', that will come to us; but, because we are spiritual beings, part of and continuous with Omnipresent, Creative Spirit, and the creative instrument is Mind, the thought we hold *at the back of our minds* will tend to materialise.

"To-night, and in future, will you, please, pray again? —but differently. You may kneel, if you like; it isn't necessary, but, since we are in His Presence, it is good manners. You will 'ask' for nothing. But, realising His Presence and Nature—as shown by Christ—you will *accept*, with grateful and radiant certainty, His provision *already made*. Then, knowing by faith that (Spirit being real), such provision is an actual, already existing fact, you will exultingly look for its materialisation. If you hear the postman . . . run to the door . . . he may have news of the job. If anyone knocks . . . race to see who it is . . . he has probably come to engage your J."

Beginning to grasp, at length, what was required, Mrs. M. promised to do as directed.

Eight days later J. rang up, his voice a-quiver with emotion: "Doctor," he managed to stammer out, "I've got my old job back, in the service!" And he has been in it now for nearly three years.

"Is my ear heavy that it cannot hear; or my hand shortened, that it cannot redeem?"

Never give in! And never give way to weakness. God's POWER does work through human FAITH. Faith, qualified by doubt, misgiving, or unbelief, is fear; but fear, qualified by belief, is FAITH. Either is almost certain to be interpreted, correspondingly, in this physical seeming environment.

"To him that believeth, all things are possible."

Mark IX, 23.

MEDIATION.

Discerning compassion, Divine Love, and faith are of the very substance of wholeness. So bring them to bear. Deny, with unwavering intensity of instructed enlightened conviction, all power or reality in outward apparent disharmonies. Affirm, with exalted thanksgiving, the inward perfection. Inspire trust. Reassure. Instil conviction of Truth. In high consciousness, speak the word of authority!

Do these persistently. Get others to help—the more batteries in circuit the mightier the Power. Teams must be formed to work in this field. Many already exist, and great victories are won.

Patience, firmness, discretion and tact will be called for to wean from deep-rooted fears and stubborn beliefs those struggling in their earlier "times." But suffering is the refiner's fire, and God and Nature are on our side.

IV. DIVINE HEALING

It is recorded that, when the Divine, Healing, Health-radiating, Vital, Loving, Life Spirit was perfectly incarnate in the Lord Jesus Christ, "great multitudes followed Him, and He healed them all."

They received their healing on three conditions:

1. *They came to Him for it*. There is not one instance on record of any "incurable" sufferer being healed who did not come to Him for it, either themselves or by proxy.
2. *They accepted His healing, by faith*, when He gave it them; thenceforward acting on the assumption of wholeness.
3. *They were to go and sin no more*. The ingenuousness must surely be self-evident of expecting Divine Spirit to heal, while we continue thinking, eating, or doing the things that make people ill.

No other conditions were imposed. The Divine Indwelling Spirit did not enquire, or care, to what religious or political beliefs they subscribed, or whether they had any or none. Faith and obedience were all that was asked. And the Universal Spirit that healed of old is the same that heals today. "Jesus Christ, the same yesterday, and today, and for ever."

SPIRITUAL SUBTERFUGE.

"All things whatsoever ye pray and ask for, *believe* that ye *have received* them and ye shall have them."

Mark XI, 24.

So taught "the man, Christ Jesus"; and, in so teaching, resorted to subterfuge. Those with whom He had to do knew nought of the workings of mind, and wot not that Spirit existed. So His problem was to inveigle infantile consciousness into productive mental alignment.

To believe we have received is to believe we already have. For example: to believe we have received and therefore already have good health is to know ourselves well and whole. Exultingly to hold in mind the unqualified assurance of already existing perfection, is to set the mental creative thought forces developing it outwardly.

Note that the Lord Jesus did not say *when* we should have! And so our Lord persuaded apprehension into *knowing the truth*; and the Truth then, as now, set men free.

He transcendently appraised what is hidden from human eyes—the Oneness of Spirit and the inborn perfection of man's true Spiritual SELF. So ineffable was His consciousness of *identity* with the Life Spirit, the Father, the Christ within, that He was able to raise the awareness of others into the realm of absolute truth, which was instantly manifest.

What He did, we in degree can do; and what His Spirit achieved in those days, is achieved in measure, today.

THE REAL OBJECTIVE.

Since defective spiritual response is the ultimate root of all ill, our true objective must be to help others as well as ourselves to better relationship with the Spirit of "Wholiness" within. Healing will naturally ensue, when relationship is adequate.

Latent within are unlimited Power—Spirit, and the creative instrument—Thought. We may do with them much what we please. Consciousness shades off through the sub- conscious to unity with all mind. And so, veiled but expectant within, are all wisdom, knowledge, and understanding, and the record of every event, past and to come. Limit, there is none; save such as is set by carnal or mental restriction. We *are* our consciousness.

PERSEVERING OBEDIENCE, HOLY ASPIRATION, and SILENT MEDITATION, will enable us to become the greater servant.

Ask, seek, knock. Deny oneself, take up one's cross, and follow HIM — CHRIST, the SPIRIT OF GOD in relation to human consciousness.

10. Illustrative Examples

1. *T. J.* is a butcher, 65 years of age, pale, flabby, and out of condition. At 4 a.m. one Friday he ran a skewer into his hand. Thirty hours later, hand and arm were swollen to double their size, with livid streaks back and front. Glands at elbow and armpit were tender and swollen; with temperature over 103.

Acute blood poisoning? Certainly. Caused by germs? Certainly. But once again, it isn't the germs that matter but that upon which they prey.

So T. J. was sent home thus to carry out detoxication, as thus:

1. No food whatever, on peril of his life. Plenty of water with orange juice.
2. As large an enema as possible, immediately; another that evening. An heroic dose of salts in the morning, followed by another enema.
3. The patient to rest, hand raised, with cold packs to his arm.

Twenty-four hours later all inflammation had gone; and the following day he returned to his work. Those who have seen doctors "fighting germs" under similar circumstances will appreciate.

2. *Mrs. S.* was in bed. Her heart was bad. Two highly competent medical men said her goitre was the *cause* of the trouble; and the only hope of recovery was operation. Incidentally, though she had been operated upon no less than five times previously for various symptoms, she was still waiting in vain to enjoy good health—not unnaturally, since she continued to live unhealthily.

Searching in the sufferer's mind and her manner of living for the true cause, a violent and consuming resentment was unearthed; while the physical toxaemia consequent upon long-continued over-indulgence in denatured foods, and insufficient outdoor exercise, was obvious.

Mrs. S. is a very fine type. She readily replaced her not unnatural resentment with generous feelings and love; and a fast of nine days was succeeded by another, self-inflicted, on water almost exclusively, of thirty-two days. The goitre gradually disappeared. The heart completely recovered. And today, four years later, Mrs. S. gives authority for stating that she is in better health than ever. The cost was three pounds.

3. **Miss S.** is 26 years of age. She had recently left hospital, where her appendix and gall-bladder were removed. It was not long before she was admitted again with acute middle-ear suppuration, for which her ear drums were perforated; and she was threatened with the "radical mastoid operation."

Previously she had undergone a double antrum operation *four times*; and had had her tonsils removed *no less than eight times*. Her medical adviser, noting her biting her nails, said she was highly strung, and prescribed *stout and cigarettes* to "steady her nerves."

4. **A man** complained of his health slipping. His advisers, after the usual fruitless search, *in his body*, for the cause, told him he was run down, and gave him a "tonic."

This made him worse.

Inquiry disclosed that he had existed on boarding house diet for eight years; and recently, with the object of bettering his position, had been in the habit of studying till late at night.

To pick himself up, he had taken two patent drug "remedies." These, for a while, had seemed to do good. But only for a while.

Unaware, like all orthodox medical men, of the nature and real causes of ill-health, his doctor had prescribed a "tonic" which consisted of:

Bromide, Strychnine, Arsenic, Chloroform, and Luminal. Five deadly poisons, which the victim was expected to swallow to "cure" the effects of overwork, bad food, and drug poisoning. [Most of the current prescription drugs in use today are considered safe and effective of course!, S.A.H.B.]

5. Twelve months ago, **Mrs. K.** had a "collapse" (due to an emotional upset). Since then, she has drunk ninety-two bottles of "medicine" at 5/6 each. This is not nearly a record. Fear and resentment were written all over her; but half an hour's reasoning sufficed to induce a changed outlook.

6. **D. T.** had a discharging malodorous cancer on his back. It had twice been treated with radium; and he was now told that "nothing more could be done."

Four months on an eliminating dietary, suitable Herbal remedies, and two consultations, completely healed the cancer; and D. T. is back in his job.

7. Recalling the premise that, whatever our symptoms may be, the cause will almost always be found under one or other or both of two primary headings, the case of **E. S.** is instructive.

E. S. is a young farmer. A few months ago, a long period of increasing digestive disorder culminated in severe abdominal pain, sleeplessness, and nervous prostration.

True to form, his advisers sought *in his body* for the cause of his troubles. They did not find it. But after eleven guineas' worth of X-Rays, they discovered a gastric ulcer or imagined they did), which they said was the *cause*. An operation, they said, was the only cure.

Applying the tests of our premise, it was found that E. S.'s breakfast consisted of porridge, chop or steak and two eggs, sauce, white toast, marmalade, and tea. Lunch: cold meat, pickles in quantity, white bread and butter, and more tea. Dinner, he "did himself proud": roast, potatoes and vegetables, with starchy puddings, much sugar and cream, and tea. In addition, he had morning and afternoon tea, with toast, hot scones, or cake; and supper of tea and biscuit and cake. He bolted his meals, and lived in a frenzy of anxiety and overwork. AND, he smoked *twelve ounces* of tobacco a week.

A tentative suggestion that the above might possibly have some bearing, brought almost instant enlightenment. With good humoured contrition, he admitted that ignorance and gluttony were the real *cause* of his misery. The ulcer was one result.

He loyally co-operated; and revision of outlook, diet, habits, and tobacco consumption, produced an astonishingly rapid, and permanent, recovery.

His X-Ray "examination" was completely unnecessary, as ninety per cent of them are [The situation is no better in the current era with MRI imaging, etc, S.A.H.B.]; and the few shillings his common-sense "treatment" cost, were made good many times over in reduced expenditure on tobacco and food.

8. **Mrs. N.** was three months pregnant. For two months she had been troubled with vomiting, which had become worse, and

worse, and worse, until finally she could not keep down even a sip of water. She had lost two and a half stone in weight. "Hyperemesis gravidarum" is the orthodox cognomen for this mild subconscious aberration.

Half an hour's "positive superimposure" enabled this young mother to eat, the same evening, a supper of hot buttered toast, crayfish, and mashed bananas and cream.

In a letter received two days later, the "patient" stated that her "stomach had completely settled down, and all that was left was a little soreness, which she supposed she must expect after two months' incessant vomiting."

The cause, was a subconscious expectation of sickness, associated in so many minds with pregnancy. Fulfilled, the expectation became foreboding; then fear; then panic, self-pity, and absolute conviction. All that was necessary was to restore confidence in wholeness — which, after all, was only the truth.

Many disordered conditions are due to a mistaken belief in the subconscious mind; and, often, considerable ingenuity will have to be displayed in outwitting the patient's misguided critical faculty.

9. An emotional **_young lady_** of nineteen summers had been "treated" for "colitis." That is to say her diet had been carefully deprived of the vitamins and minerals, lack of which is so often a causative factor; while she was being "treated" with poisonous vaccines and drugs. After ten months she was informed by two orthodox doctors and a "specialist" that "nothing more could be done," and that there was absolutely no hope. There isn't, with methods like that. The strongest could not withstand such assaults.

However, six months on unrefined foods, plus a determined health-consciousness, restored her completely to health.

10. **Mrs. R.** was sixty-eight. She had gall-stones; and her heart was too bad to allow operation. She was placed in the care of a nurse who has made Nature Cure methods a study. After six weeks on an eliminating dietary, an acute reaction, or "healing crisis" occurred. She was very ill indeed for some days with purging and vomiting. During this period she passed over seven hundred stones.

Seen three months later—*for the first time*—the lady gave every appearance of very good health.

11. **J. J.** was diagnosed with "chronic Bright's disease" (an older classification of nephritis or kidney inflammation), and had been told by specialists that he was a "spent force" and that "nothing could be done for him." But in the sixth week after adopting Nature Cure foods he duly staged the predicted "crisis." He became suddenly very ill, and was in considerable pain. He fasted—was far too ill to do otherwise—and began to pass small stones from his waterworks. He got rid of a handful. Six weeks later another "attack" occurred, during which he passed another half handful, including one large one. Following this, his health steadily improved. Seen, *for only the second time*, after a lapse of seven months, his blood pressure which had been 265, had fallen to 132; and today J. J. is a very active and dynamic force indeed, and likely to remain so for long years to come.

12. **A. B.** was twenty-three. He was committed to an asylum through losing his grip when his brother died. This was the precipitating, but not the primary cause.

Deterioration was rapid. Brought home twelve months later to die, he was reduced to a skeleton, pale as a ghost, poisoned to death, besprinkled with sores, and not one rational chink of approach remained to the shattered mentality of a now gibbering lunatic.

But "God's Power works through our faith"; and it is "patients who have to be healed, not disease."

An eliminating dietary of milk alone, first, then milk, fruit and vegetables, was adopted. Daily large enemas were administered. And faith, looking past the outward appearance, steadfastly held to the Truth of inward perfection.

The sufferer's subconscious mind was continuously impressed, direct, by the word of authority; and his belief in abnormality was unwaveringly combated.

Improvement was slow to begin with, and fluctuated for a time. But, eight months later, a gain of two and a half stone in weight, and mental grip completely regained, attested the worth of faith and obedience. And the fine soul mainly responsible is laughed at because she is "unqualified."

The cause of the boy's trouble?:—Wrong thinking, wrong feeding, and wrong habits. Fear of the consequences of sex perversion by one in a post of trust; food poisoning, due to ignorance and indifference—made much worse in "hospital"; and constipation.

13 **Mrs. P.**, seventy-four years old, was in a parlous condition of physical ill-health and mental depression. She had swallowed enough "medicines" to stock a small shop; and, after much expensive "treatment," had been told "nothing further could be done."

The true cause of her plight—her aged husband was fretting out the evening of his days in an asylum.

Pathos made compassion easy; a little comfort, teaching, and love, met with ready response and wrought a complete change in mental outlook. Transformation duly followed; and a year later she wrote:

> The neighbours marvel as I go swinging by up the hill. I never have ache nor pain; and how thankful I am to God, as I contrast my singing heart of today with my tear-stained pillow of a year ago.

When a doctor says "Nothing can be done for you," bear in mind that his opinion is probably based upon a wrong premise. Many a patient has been cured by Nature after being told that.

You may be unlucky when a doctor says he cannot do anything for you; but it is when he says he can that it is wise to beware.

Many hundreds of examples could be appended; but (by way of tempering unphilosophical optimism), think upon Lindlahr's dictum:

Though there are no diseases that are incurable, there are many patients who are.

Life has its cosmic dependency; and cosmic vibrational polarization is sometimes hereditarily (and for other reasons) so weak as to make metabolism, even with best thought and intent, subnormal or physically inefficient.

"In the case of those unfortunates who are totally or partially incapacitated for life, due to organic, muscular, bone or neural, permanent deficiency or deformity, the true physician can often do much, in the realms of mind and spirit, to develop and relieve; for spiritual evolution is not necessarily delayed or defeated by physical defect; it is, in fact, often intensified through physical restriction permitting and even enforcing greater concentration upon higher spiritual-mental opportunities.

"Acceleration of the present epoch—in life speed and greater sensitivity DEMANDS that the more sensitive type now rapidly evolving shall be extra careful in outlook and habit." (L. E. B.)

In canvassing the probable reaction of his colleagues to some of the statements above, the author anticipates a shock to some, a protest from a few, but, dawning on the countenance of the great majority comprising those most worth while, a dry grin matching the twinkle in his own eye as he envisages a change of ground to include in our armamentarium much that will immensely enhance its effectiveness.

11. The Healing Spirit Made Manifest

"Let this mind be in you, which was also in Christ Jesus: who, being IN THE FORM OF GOD, thought it not robbery to be equal with God."

Philippians II, 5 & 6.

A little over nineteen hundred years ago there came to this earth One in Whom was perfectly individualised and incarnate the attributes and resources of the Divine Creative Life Spirit.

The Lord Jesus Christ made the supreme sacrifice of coming down from His high estate to a world He knew would reject Him and despise His message, in order to show by His life and teaching the relationship between Spirit and Flesh — the Nature of God, and some of the possibilities of man.

Having triumphed finally over the weaknesses, failings, and limitations of the human physical nature, the Light of Truth was able to shine in Him in its fullness.

When the time came to begin His task, He had to decide how best to convince the people of His Divine identity. Thrusting aside human promptings, He saw it could be done in only one way: —

By subordinating His individuality to Universal Spirit the Father, God — so completely that the Father's will and purpose might find perfect expression through His individuality.

And so He was able to live without blemish; and went about healing, and teaching, and doing good.

But though He was the very Spirit of Love, He was no weak sentimentalist. While He never resented the vicious threats to

Himself, and valued Truth far above physical life, He never failed to challenge and denounce hypocrisy and exploitation by the orthodox pundits of His day. None who read Matthew XXIII can ever forget His blistering invective.

His indignation ever flamed against all who abused their authority to blind the people and batten on their miseries. And how they hated Him for it!

"And the scribes and chief priests sought *how they might destroy Him*, for they feared Him; because all the people were astonished at His doctrine."

Mark XI, 18.

Contemplating the doings of the money sharks in the temple, rising anger busied itself toying with a piece of cord. Seeing that His hands had subconsciously fashioned a whip, cold fury leaped into deadly action, and lashed avaricious shanks. . . .

"And when He had made a scourge of small cords, He drove them all out of the temple, and poured out the changers' money; and overthrew the tables.

"And said unto them, It is written, My house shall be called the house of prayer; but ye have made it a den of thieves.

"And the blind and the lame came to Him in the temple, and He healed them.

"*And when the chief priests saw the wonderful things that He did*, and the children crying in the temple, and saying, Hosanna to the son of David, *they were sore displeased*. And said unto Him, Hearest thou what these say? And Jesus said unto them, Yea: have ye never read, Out of the mouths of babes and sucklings thou hast perfected praise?"

These cruel tyrants, too cowardly to attack in the open, incited the people He came to save, to do their fell work. Forsaken by His friends, betrayed, cursed, reviled, hated, and spat upon, tortured, and doomed to a felon's death, never for an instant did His serenity falter, save when, momentarily, on the cross, He was overwhelmed by the black abyss of human antagonism.

But the Light of Love broke through, transfiguring and eternal, and the triumph of GOOD was writ for all time .. . in letters of blood.

Are we to suppose that HE who went through so much for our sakes has forgotten "His friends"? I trow not.

HE—the very Spirit of comradeship and good fellowship, of compassion and tenderness, of wit and good humour, of fierce loyalty and utter dependability: merry or sad, grieved or gay, the very incarnate soul of wisdom, knowledge, understanding and love—forget us? ... ears attuned may still hear His voice. . . .

"Not every one that saith unto ME, Lord, Lord, shall enter the Kingdom of heaven; but *he that doeth the will of my Father which is in heaven.*

"He that hath my commandments, *and keepeth them,* he it is that loveth me.

"If ye *keep my commandments,* ye shall abide in my love; even as I have kept my Father's commandments, and abide in His love.

"This is my commandment, That ye love one another, as *I have loved you.*

"He that believeth on me, the works that I do shall he do also; and greater works than these shall he do. . . ."

"I AM WITH YOU ALWAY, EVEN UNTO THE END OF THE WORLD."

We who want to help, in this great Japhetic Epoch or Gentile "world" crisis, must reflect upon His way of facing a similar state of affairs in the corresponding Hebrew or Semitic Epoch of nineteen hundred years ago.

And so, if we deny ourself, take up our "cross," and walk with Him, the Father's will and purpose may find expression, in increasing measure, through *our* individuality also, each in his own particular sphere.

12. The Standard Diet

IF it be true that mind and body are profoundly influenced by what we think, it is no less true that body and mind are greatly affected by what, when, and how we eat.

Gross feeding makes gross people; progressive nicety and simplification in eating cleanses the body, and lightens texture, so increasing spiritual sensitivity. And the more Spiritual we become, the less and the lighter the food we need. With many, eating is mostly another bad habit of mind!

The assorted appetites may be regarded as scratching posts for sharpening our spiritual claws. Where there is positive there is also negative. How should we develop self-control, or any other of the higher attributes, if there were no opportunity for practising them? We learn to master temptation by rightly exercising free will. Right feeding is both consequent upon, and conducive to, higher unfoldment.

In order to avoid long and possibly confusing explanations, which may be studied in works devoted specially to diet, the meals have been set out in such a way as to make suitable combination of foods automatic if directions are obeyed.

The writer desires to acknowledge his great debt to those of the Nature Cure School, in all countries, who for long years have battled for truth against a weight of ignorance, apathy, and antagonism, that have daunted and still daunt too many.

RULES OF EATING.

1. EAT ONLY WHEN HUNGRY. Never eat simply because it is meal time. If you don't feel genuinely hungry for a meal, MISS IT OUT.

2. EAT NO REFINED FOODS.
3. EAT SLOWLY. Chew thoroughly; specially starchy foods. See that teeth are adequate.
4. NEVER OVEREAT. Overeating is taking any food not actually needed by the body; and is one of the most prolific of all causes of disease.
5. NEVER EAT BETWEEN MEALS.
6. DON'T DRINK WITH MEALS. If thirsty, drink half an hour before, or two hours after meals.
7. ENSURE QUIET, BOTH OF BODY AND MIND. DIGESTION IS INTERFERED WITH BY ACTIVITY OF EITHER. [No doubt that Dr Williams would have been horrified by the concept of 'takeaways' and food on the go, S.A.H.B.]

BREAKFAST.

Fruit is recommended for breakfast not for its food value so much as for its vitamins and neutralising alkalinising qualities. Two kinds of fresh fruit, with one sweet dried fruit, such as dates, prunes, figs, raisins, are advised. A few nuts may be eaten as well if liked. A cup of milk may also be taken, to be SIPPED SLOWLY; but it is not necessary unless heavy manual labour is your lot. In winter the milk may be made into cocoa, or coffee substitute drink.

Occasionally for variety, stewed fresh fruit, or dried fruits, soaked for 24 hours, then raised to a convenient temperature, may be taken with milk.

Children should have milk raw, never boiled, every day.

For those who, owing to the exploitation practised under the iniquitous economic system, cannot afford the luxury of fruit, the best substitute is porridge made from coarse unrefined wheatmeal or oatmeal, and milk. On a specially cold day, it may be served once in a while instead of fruit, for all.

Do not fear under-feeding. Two meals a day have been proved sufficient. Even children are better on two meals a day than three.

LUNCH.

At this meal uncooked vegetables of all kinds should form the principal part. There is no need to keep to the general idea of salads; use your ingenuity. Recipes for salads will be found in the book, but these need not limit originality. Besides lettuce, tomatoes, celery, radishes, etc., raw shredded heart of cabbage is often used; or spinach cut finely, as well as silver beet leaves, or dandelion. All the root vegetables should be used frequently. They should be well scrubbed (not peeled or even scraped), finely shredded, and eaten raw. Use shredded carrot, turnip, swede, beetroot, and apple—in fact, any edible vegetable in any combination. They are rich in vitamin and mineral salts, and should be largely used for their purifying properties. A little grated cheese, or milled nuts, may be mixed with the salad; but on account of their fat and protein content should be used sparingly at this meal. A good nut mill may be obtained for about 3s. 6d. at most ironmongers. [Vintage nut mills can be picked up today from around US$25, S.A.H.B.]

Wholemeal bread or scones, wholemeal toast, rusks, oatcake, rye or whole wheat biscuits form the starchy part of the meal. The temptation to eat too much starch must be watched. The equivalent of from one to three slices of a two-pound loaf is enough.

A potato baked in and eaten with its jacket may be served instead of the cereal food.

Bran biscuits, wholemeal cake (very moderately), butter, and a little honey may be used; and the dried sweet fruits occasionally; but the salad should form the bulk of the meal, and starchy food used in moderation.

SUGGESTIONS FOR WORKINGMEN'S LUNCHES AND PICNICS.

During the winter any of the soup recipes will make a welcome, warming, and healthful addition to lunch. A cereal drink may be taken for variety. Either of these is easily carried in a thermos flask.

A wholemeal pie filled with any left-over vegetables, and flavoured with a little Marmite and seasoned with sage, mint, mixed herbs, curry powder, etc., is useful.

Cheese pasties, made with wholemeal flour and flavoured with onion, with or without vegetables, are also good. A little ingenuity in planning the household meals will help the housewife in preparing these lunches.

Use raisins, dates, figs, etc., freely; they are great heat and energy givers. A great variety of sandwich fillings can be improvised from raw grated vegetables, cheese, eggs, nuts, dried fruits, and combinations of these with salad dressings and mayonnaise. (See sandwich section.)

In warm weather, instead of using soup, set the vegetables into moulds, which are easily handled and carried. Suitable recipes will be found in this book. Plenty of salads should be used, not necessarily cut. Whole lettuce leaves, radishes, spring onions, carrots, etc., are easily packed and carried in a screw-topped glass jar.

DINNER.

Meat or fish are best taken only once a week. Men engaged in heavy manual work may take it oftener. Proteins in the form of eggs, cheese, or nuts, will be required in the place of meat, and suitable recipes will be found under the headings of Savoury Meat Substitute, and Egg Dishes. A variety of vegetables should be included at this meal. Always serve at least one green vegetable such as spinach, cabbage, silver beet leaves, turnip tops, string beans, leeks. Root vegetables and onions may be freely used. More sparing use should be made of peas, potatoes, dried beans, split peas, and such, on account of their high starch content. Potatoes should be cooked in, and eaten with their jackets.

All vegetables should be cooked conservatively, or steamed. Cabbage, spinach, etc., should be thoroughly washed, broken into small pieces, put into a saucepan and half to one cup of boiling water added; shake the pan frequently and the greens will cook perfectly, absorbing all, or nearly all of the water. All liquid that is left after cooking any vegetables should be taken either as a drink between meals, or used as the base for gravies or soups. This eliminates the waste of dissolved vegetable salts, purifying juices and food values, inseparable from the old method of cooking. Soda is never used, as it destroys the natural mineral salts. Salt is not used during cooking, but may be added sparingly at table. Do not use vinegar; it is a chemical preservative, not a food. Condiments also are best avoided; they are irritants.

If a pudding be included in the meal, use discrimination as to ingredients. For example, if the first part of the meal contains a substantial meat, or meat substitute dish, it is desirable to serve only a light sweet, such as stewed fruit, baked apple, with or without junket. If the first course has been very light, for example, either stuffed tomatoes, turnips, or onions, cauliflower and cheese sauce, etc., etc., something more substantial may be served: a wholemeal pudding either steamed or baked, or an egg custard.

A little cream is allowed occasionally; but white sugar NEVER. Use raw sugar only; and the less the better.

The use of baking powders, cream of tartar, baking soda, and chemical essences for flavouring is not recommended.

While a number of recipes has been included, which it is hoped will prove useful, there is scope for originality. Provided the general principle be adhered to, a great many of your favourite dishes may be adapted.

A diet sheet, showing menus for a week, suitable for any ordinary household is included.

SUGGESTED DIET FOR ONE WEEK.

Begin each day with a large, warm lemon drink. The juice of half a lemon in a large tumblerful of hot water. It is better taken unsweetened, but a little honey may be used if necessary.

1st DAY

BREAKFAST:
Grape-fruit dressed with honey. Apples, and a few dates.

LUNCH:
Everyday salad, as in recipe section. Plain Mayonnaise dressing. Wholemeal bread or toast, or scone. Bran biscuit. Butter, cheese, a little honey. Fig meat.

DINNER:
Vegetable Roast. Onion rings; creamed sprouts; grated carrot,

just heated through in oven, not cooked. Stewed raisins, junket, a little cream.

2nd DAY

BREAKFAST:

Stewed prunes, as many as required and a glass of milk; to be slowly sipped.

LUNCH:

Lentil Soup. Lettuce and celery. Cheese, butter, honey, bran biscuits, wholemeal toast.

DINNER :

Onion Soufflé. Cauliflower, mashed parsnips. Baked custard and stewed dried apricots.

3rd DAY

BREAKFAST:

Oranges and pineapple dressed with honey. Milk; to be sipped slowly after the fruit is eaten.

LUNCH:

Carrot Au Gratin. Winter salad. Wholemeal cake. Raisins.

DINNER:

Steamed fish. Marrow savoury, Brussels sprouts, or spinach. Maple walnut sponge.

4th DAY

BREAKFAST:

Plums if in season, or any fresh fruit. Stewed figs.

LUNCH:

Combination Salad and dressing of oil and lemon juice. Steamed wholemeal pudding.

DINNER:

Almond cutlets. French beans. Beetroot in butter. Date custard.

5th DAY

BREAKFAST:

Any fresh fruit in season. Junket and cream.

LUNCH:

Radishes, spring onions, celery, lettuce, cheese, butter, bran biscuits, wholemeal rusks, creamed cucumber.

DINNER:

Roast lamb; green peas, marrow, string beans. Junket, stewed prunes, cream.

6th DAY

BREAKFAST:

Melon dressed with a little ground ginger and raw sugar.

LUNCH:

Baked onion and cheese. Lettuce, etc. Wholemeal bread, cheese, butter, honey. Raisins.

DINNER:

Cauliflower roast. Grated carrots, Brussels sprouts. Eve's pudding and cream.

7th DAY

BREAKFAST:

Fruit in season. Milk.

LUNCH:

Prize tomato soup. Cauliflower and French bean salad. Toast or rusks, raisin munchers, cheese, etc.

DINNER:

Breadcrumb and onion omelette with cheese sauce, spinach, mashed parsnip, pumpkin. Dried fruit salad and cream. The Plain Mayonnaise dressing should be used with all the salads.

13. Dietary Principles For Children

So little do women today esteem the privilege of bringing God's children into the world that amenorrhoea, when not causing panic, ranks high in the list of misfortunes. Small wonder that many modern children, unwanted offspring of lust and nurtured in fear and resentment, having escaped the battery of contraceptives, abortifacients and abortionists professional and otherwise, are born deficient, epileptic, or idiot, with debased or criminal instincts.

The sins of the fathers, too (and mothers), are "visited on the children unto the third and fourth generation (of them that hate ME)."

And if fully grown bodies are susceptible to the influence of negative (and positive) thought forces, even more fruitfully so is the foetus, developing. Fret and fear, resentment and discontent, bitterness and self-pity, laziness and lasciviousness, indulgence and indolence, weakness and vile temper, too often form the thought environment of wanted as well as unwelcome children.

Drink, tobacco, and drug-sodden blood streams, defiled with emotional, food, fatigue, metabolic, and bowel poisons, convey the physical nutriment.

Mentally, morally, and physically, growth and development depend to a great extent upon an adequate supply of vitamins and mineral salts. Deficiency produces defects and deformities. When supplies are inadequate, Nature attempts to safeguard the infant at the mother's expense. If the mother does not receive enough in her food, the baby will filch his supply from her system. Destruction of teeth, obstinate debility, and premature death are outward evidence of the dangerous decay that results.

Maternal mortality has caused much concern. It need not, because appreciation of the influence of wrong thinking, wrong living, and wrong treatment, will lead to correction; and maternal mortality will then be a thing of the past.

Detailed instructions for infant feeding are not within the scope of this volume. The simpler and more natural the food the better. And the simpler and more natural the parents' mode of life, the more constant and dependable will be the natural supply. Malformations and dysfunctions of the mammary gland are among the penalties of wrong living; and inability to feed an infant on the breast must shortly become a burning disgrace.

Many babies are born overnourished, and need a period of under-feeding to compensate. Never force a baby to feed. Many a mother endures tortures at the hands of an over-zealous nurse, who, regarding the baby as a kind of machine, tries to force into him measured amounts at stated times, with little regard to his need. Many a babe who "won't take the breast," and vociferously resents attempts at compulsion, is far wiser than his supervisors.

DON'T BE AFRAID! There is every reason for confidence. Those who think, eat, and act right have little to fear from disease.

Remember the significance of Acute Illnesses. They are house-cleanings; and most of baby's untoward symptoms are explained in this way. Offspring of unhealthy parents are often born poisoned; and detoxication is to be anticipated; and is frequently the explanation of apparently untoward symptoms.

Bear in mind, also, the deleterious effect of poisons, emotional or physical, in the mother's blood. Many an infant's mysterious sickness, and even death, is caused in this way. The destructive effect of Negative Thoughts, of any description, is not confined to *our* bodies and minds; it poisons the mother's blood; it poisons her milk; but, worse still, it poisons the child's subconscious mind. The children of worrying, peevish, irritable parents are never well; and far too commonly it is the parents of sick children who need treatment, and not their unfortunate progeny.

After birth, as before, the infant, for the first few months, derives his essential vitamins and minerals from his mother. Any shortage will mean bad teeth, brittle bones, defective resistance, and generally impaired development. The mother's responsibility, both ante-natal and during lactation, should surely need no further emphasis.

When the natural supply has to be replaced or supplemented, cow's milk must be used. Ayrshire milk is the best, and Holstein next; because fat content in these is comparatively low, and the curd is soft. Milk with high fat and hard curd may need to be modified. *Never cook infant's milk.* With a pure supply, which could be easily assured, such folly amounts to a crime; while pasteurisation is a fitting monument to the false god of modern medicine.

Few indeed of the childish ailments and illnesses are unavoidable. They are mostly the direct consequence of Wrong Thinking, Wrong Feeding, and mistakes in general supervision; and are therefore a reflection upon the mother's methods. *Chicken-pox, measles, whooping-cough, diphtheria, are not diseases of childhood; they are disorders of ignorance and mismanagement.* They are not diseases at all. They are acute illnesses; and therefore reactions, curative in intent, against existing disease. If children were brought up sensibly they would never occur. Nor would "Infantile Paralysis," Tuberculosis, or other evidences of mental and food foolishness.

Immunity from disease is among Nature's rewards for obedience to her Laws. It can be had in no other way. Injection of the filthy products of animal disease into healthy bodies, to keep them well or restore them to health, is not merely self-evident folly — it brings in its train grievous retribution in the shape of dire disease. Skin, blood, and glandular disease, cancer, paralysis and insanity are among the results.

Those who refuse to think or cannot be warned deserve to be penalised. But it is hard on the child.

Much remains to be done. Better understanding and better cooperation, with adequate education in these vital matters, will progressively raise the standard.

Many adults go through a life-time of misery before they learn self-discipline. If the babe is to avoid such experience his training cannot begin too soon. We must control and develop ourselves, by cultivating, assiduously and eagerly, response to the Source of Life, in order to provide our descendants with the seemliest possible vehicles.

Let the child's thought atmosphere, from before his conception, be a glad nidus of happy assurance, joyous obedience, purity, serenity, and radiant love.

He does not, at first, know the Laws; it is for us to initiate.

Ours is the privilege. He is immensely sensitive to mental influences whether for good or ill. He responds rapidly and progressively to confidence and trust. He opens like a flower to love. He revels in happiness, peace, freedom, sunlight and air. Never over-clothe; the nude is his native state. Accustom him to react to heat and cold — his skin is his natural protector from both. Sunbathe him, naked, for a minute or two at first, and as he grows used to it, for longer periods. Sun-bathing should be done quite early in the morning; it is the light rays, not the heat rays he needs.

Feed wisely; but better ill-feed than spoil. Let him live in the open. Never let him know the smell, even at night, of stale air.

WEANING THE INFANT.

After the ninth month, or thereabouts, babies, whether fed on bottle or breast, should be introduced to solid food once a day. It should not take the form of anything other than fresh fruit or vegetables.

One of the commonest errors at this stage is to give too much starchy food; and many of the catarrhal conditions and skin eruptions are simply Nature's way of ridding the body of resulting irritant waste. The only starchy food which should be allowed at this time is occasionally a little potato. Babies cared for as recommended exhibit a gratifying freedom from fevers and so-called infective disorders.

Let the child's need be your guide. Resist the temptation in yourself and others to give sweets, cake, or unnecessary food. No one should be permitted to indulge their lack of control at the price of the child's health.

Have no misgivings! Adopt these methods for yourself and your children, and you will have the satisfaction of knowing that you are acting in accord with the findings of the most advanced food scientists all over the world.

Diet for child aged from 9 to 12 months.

Twenty-eight ounces of milk, plus 7 to 8 ounces of water, and 6 to 8 teaspoonful of sugar of milk, should be the total of 4 feeds, to be given in one day.

The milk should be increased gradually, until at 12 months 32 ounces of raw, unpasteurised cow's milk is being taken throughout the day, the 7 to 8 ounces of water having been gradually *decreased*, until at the twelfth month, the 32 ounces of undiluted, whole milk is being taken.

This is also to be the total of four feeds to be given in one day.

Between meals, throughout the day, give:

Orange juice or carrot juice, for its vitamin and mineral content, to the amount of two to four tablespoons, diluted with a little water.

At the midday meal, as well as the milk, you may give solid food in the form of ONE of the following:
1. Raw grated apple or pear. See that the fruit is fully matured and sweet. Use the skin also — very finely grated.
2. Strained tomato pulp — see also that the tomatoes are ripe and in good condition.
3. Very finely grated raw carrot; scrubbed — not peeled.
4. Steamed spinach, put through a fine sieve.
5. The floury pulp of ½ a potato, baked in its jacket.

A tablespoonful of any one of these suggestions is sufficient.

A twice-baked wholemeal crust, or rusk, on which to exercise the gums, may also be given — not for its food value, but for the help it will be to gums and teeth.

Thus, from 9 to 12 months the child will have four meals a day — three meals of plain milk, and one of milk with the addition of one or other of the suggestions given above.

Young children are better without the cereal starches so frequently advised at this time. Barley jelly, cornflour, porridge, bread and milk, mutton broth, and so on are far better left alone.

From 15 to 18 months.

A balanced dietary would now be three meals a day, mainly of milk, in much the same quantity, or a little more if the child shows a need for it, with two tablespoonful of either the fruit or vegetable suggestions given previously.

Additionally, at the evening meal, a little wholemeal bread and butter, or wholemeal toast and butter, with either a little Marmite or honey, or occasionally a little soaked dried fruit—raisins, figs, or prunes (soaked for 24 hours)—minced, and put through a sieve, is permissible.

Occasionally half a dozen dates, steamed slowly in a little milk, for a few minutes, mashed down, make a palatable spread for bread and butter; but use these dried fruits sparingly.

Later, Weet-Bix, or a similar whole grain preparation may take the place of the wholemeal bread or toast; but see that all starchy foods, all cereals, or flour foods are taken crisp and dry, never soaked in milk or gravy.

From 18 months to 2 years.

BREAKFAST: One kind of fresh fruit using any seasonable variety but not bananas (not cooked, tinned, or preserved fruit) ; and one of the sweet varieties such as a few figs, dates, or raisins.

A cup of milk may be slowly sipped after the fruit is eaten.

NO BREAD, WEET-BIX, etc., at this meal.

DINNER: Various conservatively cooked vegetables, with the addition, two or three times a week, of a small potato, baked or steamed and eaten in its jacket.

On the days when the potato is not used, a little Cottage

Cheese, or grated mild cheese may be used in addition to the vegetables.

Occasionally, instead of the cheese or potato, a lightly coddled egg may be used with the vegetables.

As an alternative suggestion, instead of the cooked vegetables, etc., one of the thick vegetable soups with whole, brown, unpolished rice may be used.

TEA: Tomato pulp or grated raw carrot as before, with either Weet-Bix, crisped in the oven and eaten cold, with a little butter, or crisp, cold, wholemeal toast, or twice-baked wholemeal bread.

The carrot, can sometimes be given as sandwiches made with wholemeal bread; and a little finely chopped lettuce and celery or other suitable vegetables may also be used.

A cup of milk may be slowly sipped after the food is eaten.

From 2 to 3½ years.

On waking, the juice of an orange.

BREAKFAST: This meal should be confined mainly to fresh uncooked fruits, with the addition of a little dried fruit and milk. Always see that fruit is ripe, thoroughly washed, and all edible skins eaten. It may be grated to ensure thoroughly mastication.

The milk must always be *slowly sipped after the fruit is eaten.*

Suggestions:
1. An orange, an apple, and a few dates, and milk.
2. Fresh ripe pears, and 3 or 4 figs (cooked or uncooked), and the milk.

3. Apples, and a dozen raisins or so (cooked or uncooked), and the milk.

Give sufficient of the fruit—mostly fresh—to satisfy hunger.

Occasionally, certainly not more than twice a week, since the object is to keep the starch content of the diet moderate, the child may have ONE of the following:

1. A little crisp, cold, wholemeal toast, and butter, with either stewed prunes, raisins, or figs; and milk.
2. Weet-Bix crisped in the oven and eaten cold, with butter and a little honey. (Do not soak the Weet-Bix in milk or other liquid). A small baked apple or a really ripe mashed banana, and milk may complete the meal.

Nothing whatever is to be taken to eat between meals (not even milk, which is a food) ; but as much water may be taken as desired. It may be flavoured with orange, lemon, or grapefruit juice. The vegetable water left over from the cooking of vegetables is an excellent drink between meals.

LUNCH: Always give at least two conservatively cooked vegetables—one green and one root; and a potato, baked or steamed and eaten in its jacket. These may be dressed with a little butter; but not made a sloppy mess with gravy, etc.

Two or three times a week, give, in addition to the vegetables, ONE of the following:
1. A little finely flaked, steamed fish.
2. An egg, very lightly boiled, poached, or coddled.
3. A tablespoonful or so of grated cheese, or Cottage Cheese.

On the days when either fish, or cheese, etc., are taken, the child will not need a second course. When vegetables and potatoes only are given, a cup of milk may be taken; and, if appetite warrants it, either a little fresh or cooked fruit; but NO CEREAL MILK PUDDINGS such as rice, sago, tapioca, macaroni, etc.

Drinks may be given throughput the afternoon if desired, as advised for the morning.

DINNER: Suggestions:
1. Any of the vegetable soups recommended; but do not use meat stock. After the soup is eaten, give *either* wholemeal bread and butter with Marmite (the bread must be at least 24 hours old, preferably 48) ; or twice-baked wholemeal bread; or crisp, cold, wholemeal toast; or Weet-Bix, with butter and Marmite. A cup of milk may be given if appetite warrants it.
2. Finely shredded lettuce and carrot, and perhaps a little shredded beetroot, or finely chopped celery — in fact, any available salad vegetables. A little grated cheese, or Cottage Cheese may also be given. A potato, or part of a potato, baked or steamed and eaten in its jacket, with a little butter. A cup of milk at this meal also.
3. Stewed fruit, junket and cream.
4. A banana, and wholemeal bread and butter; a cup of milk.
5. Dried fruits, minced if necessary; and if liked, they can be spread on the wholemeal bread and butter. A cup of milk.

Diet from 3½ to 4½ years.

On waking, and at least half an hour before breakfast, the juice of either half a lemon, orange, or grapefruit, in a large cupful of warm water. A little honey may be added for sweetening, if necessary; but no sugar.

OR

Give a cup of water, either hot or cold.

BREAKFAST:

Each of the following suggestions constitutes a meal in itself. Do not mix them, or make any alterations or additions to them. Use the suggestions in rotation.

1. An orange, or grapefruit (which may be dressed with a little honey or golden syrup, not sugar) ; or mandarins and apple; a few dates, and a cup of milk.
2. Crisp wholemeal toast, eaten cold, with butter; stewed prunes, raisins, or figs; and a cup of milk.
3. Fresh ripe pears; three or four uncooked figs; and and cup of milk.
4. Crisp, cold Weet-Bix with butter; and a really *ripe* banana.
5. Baked apple, or apples according to size, stuffed with dates; and some junket. No milk to drink.
6. Coarse oatmeal or wheatmeal porridge, with milk; and if sweetening is given, use a little honey or golden syrup, not sugar. A few dessert prunes may also be given.

No bread, porridge, or starch (cereal) of any kind is to be given at the meals which contain fresh fruit, i.e. Numbers 1, 3, and 5.

LUNCH: Always give PLENTY of conservatively cooked vegetables as before, using one green leaf variety, and two root kinds.

Every other day, with the vegetables, give *ONE* of the following:

1. An egg, lightly boiled, or coddled, or poached, or scrambled.
2. A little fresh fish, baked, boiled, or steamed. (No tinned or smoked fish).
3. A helping of Cottage Cheese.
4. Two or three tablespoonfuls of grated mild cheese.

On the days when either fish, egg, or cheese is given, do not use potatoes. Starches and proteins are best kept apart.

NO made pudding should be given.

Fresh fruit, or cooked fresh fruit may be given for dessert, if appetite warrants it; but no milk puddings, or even milk to drink, are necessary.

On the alternate days to those when the cheese, fish, egg, etc., are taken, give the vegetables as before, with the addition of a potato, baked and eaten in its jacket, dressed with a little butter.

On these days, junket and cooked dried fruit may be given. Do not use steamed puddings or cereal milk puddings meanwhile.

DINNER (or Lunch) : A salad made of shredded lettuce (or, if lettuce is scarce, young raw cabbage, or other greens such as spinach, silverbeet, watercress, etc.), celery, finely grated raw carrot, and a little white turnip and beetroot, and a few raisins. Use a dressing of cream, lemon juice, and honey, but *NO VINEGAR, PICKLES*, etc.

Cottage Cheese, or finely milled Brazil or freshly shelled walnuts may be given with the salad.

A potato, baked or steamed in its jacket, should also be given with the salad.

When salad vegetables are plentiful, sometimes give uncut lettuce, tomato, celery, radish, etc.

Use the salad or salad vegetables, with cheese, potato, etc. on the days when potato is not given at the dinner meal.

The salad should be used *three times a week*, at least; and on the alternate days, use one or other of the following suggestions, taking them in rotation:

1. Vegetable Soup — not meat stock.

   After the soup is eaten, but not with it, give *either* wholemeal bread with butter; *or* Twice-baked wholemeal bread; *or* Crisp, cold, wholemeal toast; *or* Weet-Bix crisped in the oven and eaten cold, with butter and Marmite.

   A baked apple may also be taken.

2. Stewed fruit, junket, and cream. No bread, etc.

3. A banana, and wholemeal bread and butter; and a cup of milk. A piece of plain wholemeal cake, and one or two bran biscuits.

4. Dried fruits, wholemeal bread and butter; and a cup of milk.

A cup of milk may be given after any of the above suggestions if appetite warrants it, but not otherwise.

Throughout the day, between meals, give the drinks of plain water, or flavoured with lemon, orange, or grapefruit juice as before.

Diet from 4½ to 5 years.

At least half an hour before breakfast, the juice of half a lemon, orange, or grapefruit in a cup of water, as before.

BREAKFAST: Use the following breakfasts in rotation. Do not mix them or make additions to them. Each constitutes a meal in itself.

1. One or two apples, which may be grated, if desired; one orange, and 4 to 6 dates. A glass of milk. Occasionally, the apple may be baked and stuffed with dates. This will give variety.
2. Porridge made from coarse whole wheatmeal or oatmeal. Also a really ripe banana, and a glass of milk.
3. An orange or grapefruit (dressed with honey if liked), and a dish of stewed prunes, hot or cold. A glass of milk.
4. Wholemeal toast, crisp and cold, with a little butter; 4 or 5 figs; a few dates. A glass of milk.
5. Apples, pears, and a glass of milk.
6. Weet-Bix, with butter; raisins and a glass of milk.
7. Grapes, or other seasonable fresh fruit, stewed prunes or figs; and half to one ounce of Brazil nuts, which must be well masticated. If proper mastication is not certain, grate the nuts. NO MILK.

LUNCH (or Dinner) : The following suggestions should be used in rotation:
1. Lettuce and tomato salad, baked or steamed potato, in its skin. Bran Biscuits and butter; a little honey. Use a salad dressing of cream, lemon juice and honey.
2. Wholemeal bread and butter, whole young carrots, if very well chewed, otherwise grate them; a few dates.
3. Vegetable soup, or Scotch Broth.
4. Some lettuce and tomato; crisp, cold, wholemeal toast, lightly buttered, a little honey; and a really ripe banana may also be given.
5. Sandwiches of wholemeal bread and butter, with a filling of Marmite, lettuce, and mild cheese. A piece of plain wholemeal cake.

6. A baked or steamed potato, in its skin, lettuce, tomato, and celery, or other raw salad vegetables. Stewed prunes.
7. Raw vegetable salad as before, dressed with cream, lemon juice and honey. Twice-baked wholemeal bread, crisp and cold, with a little butter. (Use grated raw roots such as carrot, parsnip, turnip, beetroot, etc., in the salad as well as the lettuce and tomato.) Junket, and apple or pear, stuffed with dates. No bread.

DINNER:

1. Onions stewed in milk, and the liquid made into wholemeal cheese sauce. Mashed pumpkin, silver-beet, or string beans when seasonable. A light wholemeal pudding, baked or steamed. One containing dried fruit, for preference.
2. Meat such as mutton or lamb (*no fried foods*); and at least two vegetables, conservatively cooked.
3. An egg, scrambled, poached or lightly boiled, with at least two kinds of vegetables as before. Stewed raisins, junket and a little cream.
4. Steamed fish, creamed carrots, spinach or cabbage. A plain baked apple. Cauliflower and cheese sauce made with wholemeal, and other seasonable vegetables such as one root and one green. Some fresh or dried fruit.
5. Casseroled poultry, cooked with plenty of suitable vegetables, and served with one green leaf kind.
6. A large raw vegetable salad, as mentioned previously, and one potato, baked or steamed and eaten in its jacket. A small helping of steamed or baked wholemeal pudding.

Throughout the day, between meals, give water, plain, or flavoured with lemon, orange, or grapefruit juice, for drinks, as before.

From 5½ to 7 years

the above dietetic instructions may be used with the following amendments:

BREAKFAST:

1. Fresh and dried fruit and milk as above; but the *yolk only* of one egg may be beaten into the milk.
2. As before.
3. Fresh fruit, and stewed prunes as above; but *instead of* the milk, half to one ounce of freshly shelled Brazils or walnuts may be used — not peanuts or chestnuts.
4. As before.
5. Fresh fruit, with Brazil or walnuts *instead of* the milk.
6. Weet-Bix, raisins, and milk as above; with the addition of a baked apple, stuffed with dates.

LUNCH (*or Dinner*) : This meal to remain as set out above.

DINNER:

1. Onions and wholemeal cheese sauce, and other vegetables as before, with the addition of a potato, baked and eaten in its jacket. The light wholemeal pudding as above.
2. Meat such as mutton or lamb, with vegetables as above; and a baked stuffed apple.
3. This meal to remain as above.
4. Steamed fish, with vegetables; and instead of the baked apple mentioned above, give either uncooked fresh fruit, or stewed dried fruit, or one of the simple fruit salad suggestions given in the recipe section.

5. Vegetables, etc., with the addition of a potato, baked or steamed, and eaten in its jacket; and some fresh or dried fruit as above.
6. Occasionally, instead of the casseroled poultry as mentioned above, liver may be given, with suitable vegetables, etc., as advised.

Plain water, or water flavoured with lemon, orange, or grapefruit juice to be given for drinks as required throughout the day, as before.

14. Fasting; Eliminative and Special Diets

IMPORTANT! *All these diets are accompanied by:*
1. VITAMIN B COMPOUNDS
2. SEAWEED POWDER
and
3. OLIVE OIL
to promote Re-mineralisation and Detoxication.

Vitamin B compounds can be obtained from preparations of wheat-germ; the vital, life-giving part of wheat discarded by "civilization" as "offals," till dead starch diet has caused disease; then brought back for sale. Other good sources are yeast extracts such as Marmite, Vegemite and Vitam-R. As long as food-massacre is allowed to continue, just so long will it be necessary to buy Vitamin B preparations, to avert the consequences.

Seaweed powder is advised because it contains, in assimilable form, minerals which the modern dead diet lacks. It is NOT a substitute for right production or selection of food. It is purely a temporary expedient.

Olive Oil is the most powerful natural detoxicating agent we possess. It is demulcent, and anti-acid. *Olive Oil is Nature's anti-toxin*. It should be freely used, both as food and medicine.

Because Calcium is not metabolised in absence of Vitamin D, Ostelin® (Vitamin D_3) is often given, specially in the winter months when sunlight is less accessible.

TYPES OF ELIMINATIVE AND SPECIAL DIETS

In presenting the following modifications of the Nature Cure method of using foods, Fasting, and Numbers One and Two, are used mainly either during Healing Crises, or, in the robust but heavily toxic, to promote and facilitate elimination.

The Milk Diet, Number Three, serves a similar purpose in weak or asthenic people, or tuberculous subjects.

Numbers Four and Five are for more prolonged use in those with systems heavily burdened with acid waste. Their good effect will be much increased by vigorous exercise.

Number Six is for patients with digestive disorder. With thorough mastication, excellent results are obtained.

Number Seven is for prolonged use by those whose toxic troubles make animal proteins inadvisable.

Number Eight is a heavy dietary, sometimes used for labourers, or those temporarily requiring a building dietary.

With all these variations, faithful observance of the directions outlined for Right Thinking and Healthy Habits is essential. Never let it be forgotten, however, that our ultimate purpose should be to grow in spiritual consciousness; to develop receptivity, responsiveness, and sensitivity; so that decreasing density and resistance may express in increasingly effective action and results.

15. Directions For Carrying Out A Fast

IT must be understood that accurate directions cannot be given which could cover all types of case. The following directions will be found of general application:

FOR ACUTE ILLNESS.
1. Give no food whatever, not even milk.
2. Give copious drinks; weak citrus fruit drinks are best; or plain water, if preferred, and plenty of it. (In cases of abdominal emergency do not even give drinks.)
3. Give a hot bath immediately.
4. Promote perspiration for half an hour, subsequently, by means of cold and hot packs or hot bottles. Then sponge the patient, and clothe in clean garments.
5. Use the enema, running in as much warm saline as the patient can contain. (Saline is water with a level teaspoonful of ordinary salt to each pint.) Let the return be made into a bed-pan. Repeat the enema every day; two or three times a day if necessary. (Do not use the enema in peritonitis.)
6. Apply a hot pack for five minutes, followed by a cold pack for one minute, to the seat of inflammation or pain. Repeat the packs two or three times, as required.
7. Whatever else is done, see that FAITH never falters, even, or specially, when the outlook seems most untoward. Miracles are worked through Faith today as 1900 years ago. Sufferers can often be brought back from the jaws of death, exceptionally even from beyond.

FOR CHRONIC DISEASE.

1. Give copious drinks: orange or lemon or grapefruit juice, well diluted with water. Vegetable water is valuable, either derived from cooking in the ordinary way, or made by simmering together for three hours, in plenty of water, as many varieties as possible of chopped vegetables (not potatoes). Bran and raisin water may be given. Soak together for six hours, in a pint of cold water, and then strain, a teacupful of bran, and a small handful of raisins. All these supply vitamins and minerals; and promote elimination.

2. Use the enema every day; run in, for an adult, two quarts, or more, of warm saline, at each administration. Let the patient lie flat, with hips on a higher level than shoulders. If returns are very profuse, use the enema twice daily. An alternative position is with the patient lying on the left side, with knees drawn up.

3. Tepid or cold bath daily; preceded by friction rub, and followed by brisk towelling.

4. Morning exercises, and deep breathing. Daily walk, as far as possible without undue fatigue.

5. Manipulative treatment, and massage, when needed.

6. A positive mental attitude is absolutely essential.

16. Eliminative and Special Diets

SEE Chapter 14 for guidance on which diet to use.

1. FRUIT DIET.
(For healing crises, etc)

Consists of three meals a day, of fresh, ripe, mature fruit, one kind only at each meal. Eat enough to satisfy hunger.

Between meals, vegetable water, with or without Marmite, may be taken.

2. FRUIT AND VEGETABLE DIET.
(For healing crises, etc)

BREAKFAST: Fresh fruit only, one kind.
LUNCH: A large salad, as suggested for the Standard Diet; dressing. NO STARCH WHATEVER.
DINNER: Cooked vegetables only.

3. MILK DIET.
(When weak or asthenic.)

On waking, and at least half an hour before the first milk is taken, drink a large glass of hot water into which has been squeezed the juice of half a lemon. It may be sweetened with a little honey.

At 8 a.m. (or earlier to suit individual convenience), and at regular two hourly intervals throughout the day, finishing at 8 p.m., take 5 ounces (150 ml) of milk. Each day, increase the amount by one ounce (30 ml) each drink (i.e. 5 ounces every two hours for the first day, 6 ounces every two hours for the second day, etc.) until one pint (20 ounces/600 ml) of milk is being taken every two hours.

If the full pint is a little too much, take the amount most easily managed. Anything over 14 ounces (400 ml) will do; though most people manage the pint easily. The milk should be beaten well with an egg-beater to ensure aeration.

The milk may be warmed, but not heated.

The milk must be sipped slowly always. It is a food, not a drink; and if swallowed in large mouthfuls will form large curds in the stomach and may cause discomfort.

Throughout the day, water may be taken to drink, according to need, between the amounts of milk.

When fruit is prescribed in addition to milk, eat one kind, three times a day, with the milk, at ordinary meal hours.

Any seasonable fruit, such as oranges, grapes, grapefruit, mandarins, pineapple, etc., may be used for variety; and, provided they are ripe and sweet, others may be added as they come into season. Use fresh fruit only. No tinned, cooked, or preserved fruit. See that the fruit is fully matured. Be sure to masticate well. The fruit should be washed carefully to remove poisonous spray; and all edible skins eaten.

Before each of these meals, a dessertspoonful of olive oil should be taken.

On going to bed, a citrus fruit drink as advised for the morning should be taken.

4. ELIMINATING DIET.

(For acid waste burden, combine diet with vigorous exercise.)

At least half an hour before breakfast, a weak, warm, unsweetened lemon drink—the juice of half a lemon in a large tumblerful of hot water.

BREAKFAST: Two varieties of fresh fruit—any seasonal kinds but not bananas. Eat sufficient to satisfy hunger. *NOTHING ELSE AT ALL*. No bread, porridge, etc.

Throughout the day, between meals, drink according to need, of plain water, either hot or cold, or flavoured with orange, lemon, or grapefruit juice, or Marmite, or vegetable water, with or without Marmite.

LUNCH (or *dinner*) : Always a *LARGE* salad, using a good variety of grated raw vegetables as mentioned in "Everyday Salad." (If lettuce is scarce, young raw cabbage, spinach, silverbeet, watercress, etc., make excellent substitutes.)

Dress the salad liberally with an olive oil and lemon juice dressing. The one recommended is either Plain or Special Mayonnaise. *NO VINEGAR, PICKLES OR CONDIMENTS*.

Occasionally, instead of a dressed salad, you may take uncut salad vegetables, such as lettuce, tomato, celery, radish, spring onion, etc.

These raw vegetables are very necessary. They supply the vitamins and minerals which the system lacks. Therefore they should form the largest part of the meal.

Take also one or two Weet-Bix, crisped in the oven and eaten cold, with a little butter; *OR* Ryvita Biscuits; *OR* a decent-sized potato, baked and eaten in its jacket, with a little butter.

DINNER: Take *PLENTY* of conservatively cooked vegetables, using always one green leaf variety and at least two other kinds each day; but do not use potatoes at this meal.

NO MEAT, etc. NOTHING ELSE.

5. REDUCING DIET.

(For acid waste burden, combine diet with vigorous exercise.)

BREAKFAST: Ripe juicy fruits—two or three varieties—choosing from those in season. Use plums sparingly, and bananas not at all. Watermelon, without sugar. may be taken when seasonable.

Eat sufficient fruit to satisfy hunger. The fruit must be ripe and fully matured. Wash the fruit well and eat all edible skins.

Take also one ounce of freshly shelled nuts—walnuts, Brazils, or pecans.

NOTHING ELSE AT ALL. No bread, no dried fruit; no porridge, no tinned, preserved, or bottled fruit.

Throughout the day, between meals, drink according to need only of plain water, hot or cold, or flavoured with either lemon, orange, or grapefruit juice, or Marmite, or vegetable water, with or without Marmite.

LUNCH (or *dinner*): Take a *LARGE* leafy salad, or tomatoes when seasonable. Do not use root vegetables in the salad meanwhile; but variety may be given by using young heart of cabbage, spinach, watercress, dandelion, endive, spring onion, sorrel, or sea kale.

Dress the salad with an olive oil and lemon juice dressing—either the Plain or Special Mayonnaise is recommended.

Take also one piece of twice-baked wholemeal bread, crisp and cold, with a little butter.

NOTHING ELSE AT ALL. No cake, pastry, meat, fish, egg, etc.

DINNER: Two or three varieties of conservatively cooked vegetables, using at least one green leaf kind each day, as well as one or two others, choosing from those in season,—not potatoes.

In addition to the vegetables, take *either*: A little lean meat (roasted, grilled, or braised) ; fresh fish (baked, boiled, or steamed, not tinned or smoked) ; OR an ounce of freshly shelled Brazils or walnuts may be either eaten whole or milled and sprinkled on the vegetables,

NOTHING ELSE; NOT EVEN BREAD, OR MILK. NO PUDDINGS.

6. DIGESTIVE DIET.
(For digestive disorders.)

At least half an hour before breakfast, a weak, warm, unsweetened lemon drink should be taken—the juice of half a lemon in a large tumblerful of hot water.

BREAKFAST: Take the juice of one orange, and half to one pint of milk. The orange juice may be added to the milk if desired. It will not curdle; or, if preferred, the orange may be eaten whole.

The milk may be warmed; not boiled, and it must be slowly sipped. *NOTHING ELSE AT ALL. NO bread, porridge, etc.*

Throughout the day, between meals, drink according to need of plain water, either hot or cold, or flavoured with orange, lemon, or grapefruit juice; or Marmite, or vegetable water with or without Marmite.

LUNCH: Use the following suggestions in rotation—one each day. Each one constitutes a meal in itself, so do not mix them or make alterations or additions to them.

1. A large potato, or two smaller ones, baked or steamed and eaten in the jacket, with a little butter, followed by a well-baked apple stuffed with dates; and half a pint of junket, with a little cream.

2. A moderate amount of wholemeal bread, which must be at least twenty-four hours old; and butter; and Marmite, with lettuce leaves.
3. One pint of milk, with the *yolks only* of two eggs beaten into it, with a little honey for sweetening, if necessary. Sip this slowly. No sugar; no essence. NOTHING ELSE AT ALL. No bread, no Weet-Bix, etc.
4. Weet-Bix crisped in the oven and eaten cold, with butter; and some dried fruit—dates, raisins, or figs.

DINNER: Two or three kinds of conservatively cooked vegetables, using always one or two green leaf varieties and one or two others, if possible, each day; but do not use potatoes at this meal.

In addition to the vegetables, take *every other day, either*:
1. Meat (roasted, grilled, or braised).
2. Fish (baked, boiled, or steamed. No tinned or smoked fish).
3. Egg or Egg Dish.

Use these in rotation.

NO BREAD, NO PUDDINGS. NOTHING ELSE.

A dessertspoon of pure olive oil should be taken a few minutes before each of these meals.

7. READJUSTING DIET.

(For toxic troubles, when animal proteins inadvisable.)

On waking, and at least half an hour before breakfast, take a weak, warm, unsweetened lemon drink—the juice of half a lemon in a large tumblerful of hot water.

BREAKFAST: Fresh fruit, two or three varieties, choosing from those in season. Use plums sparingly; and do not use bananas.

Eat sufficient fruit to satisfy hunger, making sure that it is ripe and sweet. Do not take cooked, tinned, bottled or preserved fruit. Wash the fruit well and eat edible skins.

And, in addition, take *alternately, either*:

1. Half a pint of milk, *slowly sipped after the fruit is eaten.*
2. About an ounce of freshly shelled Brazils or walnuts.

NOTHING ELSE. NO BREAD. NO PORRIDGE. NO EGG. NO TEA, etc.

Throughout the day, between meals, drink to need of water, hot or cold, plain, or flavoured with lemon, orange, or grapefruit juice, or Marmite; or vegetable water with or without Marmite.

LUNCH (or dinner) : Take a *LARGE* salad, using a good variety of grated raw vegetables as mentioned in "Everyday Salad." If lettuce is scarce, young raw cabbage, spinach, silverbeet, or other green may be used instead, as the base of the salad, with the raw roots as suggested.

Dress the salad liberally with an olive oil, honey, and lemon juice dressing. Either the Plain or Special Mayonnaise is recommended.

A little grated cheese, or Cottage Cheese, or milled nuts may be used with the salad.

Sometimes, instead of a dressed salad, uncut salad vegetables such as lettuce, tomato, celery, radish, spring onion, etc. may be taken. These raw vegetables are very necessary to supply essential vitamins and minerals. Therefore let the salad or salad vegetables form the largest part of the meal.

Occasionally, for variety, one of the cooked Vegetable Dishes may be taken. Some uncut lettuce and tomato should also be used at this meal.

In addition to the salad, raw vegetables, or Vegetable Dish, as above, take a moderate amount of *ONE* of the following:

1. A decent-sized potato, baked or boiled and eaten in the skin, with a little butter.
2. Wholemeal toast, crisp and cold, with butter.
3. Twice-baked, stale wholemeal bread, and butter.
4. One or two Weet-Bix, crisped in the oven and eaten cold, with butter.
5. Crispbread or Ryvita, or other rye or whole wheat biscuit.

Take only one of the foregoing starch suggestions each day. Do not mix them.

One or two bran biscuits, lightly buttered, may also be taken at this meal.

NOTHING ELSE AT ALL. No meat, fish, egg, tea, etc.

DINNER: Plenty of conservatively cooked vegetables, using always one green leaf variety and at least two other kinds; but no potatoes at this meal. Use any seasonable vegetables.

In addition to the vegetables, take *either*:

1. A glass of milk, slowly sipped, or Cottage Cheese; or Cheese Sauce; or grated mild cheese.
2. Cooked lima or haricot beans (well soaked — at least 24 hours beforehand), or lentils. These may sometimes be embraced in a Meat Substitute Dish.
3. Freshly shelled nuts, using either Brazils or walnuts (not peanuts or chestnuts). These must be well masticated, or if desired, they may be milled.
4. The *yolks* only of 2 eggs, either poached or beaten raw in half to one pint of milk. No sugar; no essence.

If occasionally, a Meat Substitute Dish containing either beans, lentils, or nuts is taken, an egg for binding may be used if necessary.

Occasionally, too, Omelette or Soufflé is permissible in place of the above suggestions. In this case, of course, the whole egg may be used.

The diet is to be kept entirely free of meat or fish meanwhile. Animal proteins may putrefy. This applies also to eggs; and is the reason for their somewhat restricted use. The protein content of the diet consists of natural foods, and is in sufficient quantity for present needs in the suggestions given above.

NO MADE PUDDINGS AT ALL. Use only raw or cooked fresh fruit, and junket for dessert.

Fresh fruit for stewing must be ripe and sweet so that added sugar is not required. If a little sweetening is really necessary, use honey; not sugar.

NO BREAD. NO TEA. NO CEREAL of any sort at this meal.

8. HEAVY DUTY DIET.

(For labourers, a building up diet.)

At least half an hour before breakfast, the juice of half a lemon in a large tumblerful of hot water, unsweetened, should be taken.

BREAKFAST: The following suggestions to be used in rotation. Each one constitutes a meal in itself, and should not be altered or added to. Do not mix the suggestions.
1. Two or three varieties of fresh fruit, using any seasonable varieties, but not bananas. The fruit must be fully matured and sufficient should be taken to satisfy hunger. It should be washed but not peeled; and all edible skins should be eaten.

One ounce of freshly shelled Brazil nuts or walnuts also. Masticate well. *NOTHING ELSE WHATEVER. NO BREAD. NO PORRIDGE, etc.*

2. *EITHER* wholemeal bread, at least 24 hours old; or wholemeal toast; crisp and cold; or Weet-Bix, crisped in the oven and eaten cold, with butter (do not soak these in liquid) ; and one variety of uncooked dried fruit, i.e. either 4 to 6 figs; 8 to 10 dates; or about two dozen raisins. A little honey or Marmite may also be used; and a really ripe banana may be taken. Half a pint of milk may be slowly sipped after the the food is eaten. *NOTHING ELSE WHATEVER.*

3. Junket—up to half a pint; and *EITHER* a baked apple stuffed with dates (no sugar) , or a plate of stewed prunes, raisins, or figs. One variety of fresh fruit may be eaten if necessary to satisfy hunger. If all the milk is not taken in junket form, the remainder may be drunk after the food is eaten. *NOTHING ELSE. NO NUTS*, or starch at this meal.

Throughout the day, if thirsty, drink between meals either plain water, hot or cold, or vegetable water with or without Marmite, or Marmite and water, or bran water, or water flavoured with either lemon, orange, or grapefruit juice.

LUNCH (or *dinner*) : A LARGE salad, using a good variety of grated raw vegetables as mentioned in "Everyday Salad." If lettuce is not always procurable, young cabbage, spinach, silverbeet or other green may be used, with grated roots.

Dress the salad liberally with an olive oil, honey, and lemon juice dressing—Plain or Special Mayonnaise.

A little grated cheese, or Cottage Cheese, or milled nuts may be taken with the salad.

Occasionally, instead of a dressed salad, uncut salad vegetables may be taken, such as celery, radish, spring onion, lettuce, tomato, etc., with either Vegetable Soup or a Vegetable Dish, as advised below.

The salad should be used every second day, with one of the starches (cereals) mentioned below. Do not mix these suggestions; but be content to take only one kind of starch at a meal, i.e. ONE of the following:

1. Wholemeal toast, eaten cold, with butter.
2. Twice-baked wholemeal bread, at least 24 hours old, and butter.
3. Wholemeal bread and butter.
4. Wholemeal scone, not new or hot, and butter.
5. A large potato or two smaller ones, baked or steamed in the skin with a little butter. (Eat the skin also.)
6. Weet-Bix, crisped in the oven and eaten cold, with butter.

One or two bran biscuits, or bran muffins may be used in addition to the above starch suggestions.

For variety use:

One of the Vegetable Soups, with one of the above starch suggestions. (Do not take bread, etc., with the soup; though it may be eaten afterwards.) Take also salad or salad vegetables;

OR

A savoury Vegetable Dish, with one of the above starch suggestions, and salad or uncut salad vegetables;

OR

Savoury whole brown rice in moderate quantity — natural rice cooked with sliced onion; or savoury rice and tomato.

Sweet rice such as Raisin Rice may occasionally be used for variety.

If the rice is taken, no other starch should be used; though salad or salad vegetables may be used freely at this meal.

DINNER: Always PLENTY of conservatively cooked vegetables, using two greens and one or two root kinds if possible. Any seasonable vegetables may be used.

Potatoes though fairly low in starch content, are best kept apart from animal proteins, which are meat, fish, etc.

In addition to the vegetables, as above…

ONCE a week take:

- Meat (roasted, grilled, or braised) may be used.
- Butcher's small-goods, i.e. tripe, brains, liver or kidneys, are admissible; but *not* sausages, saveloys, rissoles, or brawn.
- Fish, baked, boiled, steamed, or fried in olive oil.
- Nuts, walnuts or Brazils; or one of the Meat Substitute Dishes.
- Egg or Egg Dish.
- Grated mild cheese, Cheese Dish, Cottage Cheese, or Cheese Sauce.

On the remaining day, either cooked vegetables, as mentioned above should be taken, with a potato, or instead of the cooked vegetables, a salad as mentioned for lunch, with a potato, baked or steamed and eaten in its jacket.

When taking meat or the butcher's small goods, only fresh raw fruit, or cooked fresh or dried fruit, with a little cream, should be used for dessert.

On the days when fish, or an egg or egg dish are taken, junket or baked custard, or one of the light puddings of the Spanish Cream variety, with cooked fresh fruit and a little cream, or raw fruit, may be taken.

Puddings containing rice, sago, etc., should not be used with any of the above suggestions; though a light steamed wholemeal pudding, or a rice pudding made with natural, whole brown unpolished rice may be used on the day when the vegetable meal, with either grated cheese, Cheese Sauce, Cottage Cheese, or nuts or a potato is taken, as suggested.

17. Breaking The Fast

AFTER fasting, fruit meals should be given for a day, or days, according to the length of the fast. For example: fruit meals for one day when breaking a short fast of eight to ten days. Three days on fruit meals after fasting for fourteen to twenty days; and so on. Eat one kind of fresh ripe fruit, not bananas, at each meal. After short fasts of two or three days, feeding is then resumed — eating less to begin with. After the necessary fruit days, proceed as follows:

1st Day:
BREAKFAST: Fresh fruit, one or two kinds.
LUNCH: Cut lettuce and tomato, with a little shredded raw carrot.
DINNER: One cooked green vegetable (spinach, string beans, etc.).
Begin and end the day with a weak warm lemon drink. Between meals, drinks as while fasting.

2nd Day:
BREAKFAST: Two kinds of fresh fruit.
LUNCH: Salad of lettuce and tomato, with raw shredded carrot, turnip, and beetroot. Oil, or cream and lemon dressing.
DINNER: Two cooked green vegetables (spinach, beans, silver beet, asparagus, etc.).

3rd Day:
BREAKFAST: Two kinds of fresh fruit; and one dried, such as figs, dates, muscatels, raisins.

LUNCH: Salad as before, with other grated raw vegetables, pieces of banana, sultanas, etc. A potato baked and eaten with its jacket; a little butter.

DINNER: Three cooked vegetables.

4th Day:

BREAKFAST: As before.

LUNCH: Salad as before. Three or four Weet-Bix, and butter.

DINNER: Poached egg on spinach. Stewed prunes and cream.

5th Day:

BREAKFAST: Fruit as before.

LUNCH: Salad of any variety. Two or three pieces of twice baked bread, and butter. Two or three bran biscuits, with butter and honey.

DINNER: Steamed fish, or roast mutton, with two or three vegetables, not potato. Baked apple, with date filling; a little cream.

6th Day:

BREAKFAST: As before; a few walnuts, or brazil nuts may be added.

LUNCH: A cooked salad, with dressing, and Cottage Cheese; two pieces of wholemeal toast and butter.

DINNER: One of the Meat-Substitute Dishes, three vegetables; a date custard.

From now on, follow the Standard Diet. Stick to the principle, but use your imagination. Don't *fuss* over food; it would be better to eat much rubbish than to be continually concerned about what you have.

The effect upon the acute suppurative conditions of fasting and general eliminative procedures is often dramatic. Whitlows (inflammatory reactions of the fingers) disappear; abscesses often absorb; poisoned hands, limbs, or feet, with acute lymphangitis and lymphadenitis, recover as if by magic. Suppurative conditions of antrum, sinus, and mastoid, respond more gradually, but almost equally satisfactorily. Osteomyelitis, both acute and chronic, recovers in a way never dreamed of by orthodoxy. Appendicitis, salpingitis, peritonitis, and almost every other "itis," the same.

18. Suggestions For Hotel Diet

PROGRESSIVE managers everywhere are beginning to cater for those reluctant to destroy themselves with wrong food. Seek such, and encourage them. Meanwhile, even where meals follow most orthodox lines, much may be done to minimise punishment.

ON RISING IN THE MORNING, take a large weak citrus fruit drink; or simply two or three glasses of plain water. No biscuits or tea.

BREAKFAST: One or more kinds of fresh fruit, eaten with skins if edible. In addition, one kind of dried fruit; either a few nuts, or a glass of milk, slowly sipped. If fresh fruit is unobtainable, dried fruits are usually, to be had, either cooked or uncooked; and these, together with nuts or junket or milk, are quite enough.

An orange or two, almost always available, and half a pint of milk, slowly sipped, make an admirable breakfast.

DO NOT EAT ANYTHING ELSE WHATEVER.

LUNCH: Most hotels, and restaurants, will provide Salad Vegetables; but few have any idea of the quantity required. With a little good-humoured explanation, this difficulty may usually be overcome.

If salad vegetables are not forthcoming, buy them and eat them elsewhere, in variety and quantity. DO NOT USE VINEGAR, OR CUCUMBER, etc. FLOATING IN VINEGAR.

Insist upon wholemeal bread, toasted if desired; or Weet-Bix, or other whole-wheat or rye biscuit.

Butter, cheese and Marmite, are desirable. A few dried fruits are permissible, as well as honey.

In the winter, soup may be taken as well.

DINNER: Remembering that vegetables should form the bulk of our diet, bargain for all you can get.

For protein, eat meat, fish, poultry, or egg dish (omelette, etc.)

Sweets would be best left alone; but if you insist, junket, baked custard, or one of the usually available light puddings of the Spanish Cream or Fruit Shape order should be selected.

Avoid bread, pastry, floury puddings, cakes, rich or spicy sauces and gravies, condiments, etc.

Don't be afraid of being half starved. Learn to accommodate consumption to need.

WHEN THE PEOPLE DEMAND SENSIBLE FEEDING THE DEMAND WILL BE MET.

19. Hints on Preparation and Cooking

VEGETABLES should be fresh. They should be well washed and scrubbed, not peeled or even scraped, for it is in the skin and very near the surface that most of the minerals are found.

The best method of cooking is to steam them; otherwise cook in as little water as possible and save whatever is left of the water after the cooking process is completed, and use either to drink, or as the base for soups, sauces, gravies, etc.

Soda should never be used in the cooking of any vegetable, and salt should only be added during the last minute of the cooking process; better still, cook without using salt and add a little at table. Vegetables take very much less time to cook if salt is not used. In any case 15 minutes is sufficient for almost all vegetables.

Green vegetables such as cabbage are best shredded somewhat finely, and then plunged into about a cupful of boiling water, cooked for 10 to 15 minutes, drained, and chopped, and served with a little butter. Reserve the water.

Root vegetables are best put into cold water, brought to boiling point, and then gently simmered for 15 minutes. The water left over may be turned into sauce (only very little should be used, and with a tablespoonful of butter added, the vegetables will not burn), and served with them.

Two or three root vegetables, diced and cooked together make a pleasant change.

Vegetables such as lettuce, string beans, cabbage, cauliflower, if wrapped closely in paper will keep fresher.

Vegetables should not be soaked in water for any longer than is absolutely necessary to draw out small insects and grubs. Too many of the mineral salts are wasted if care is not taken about this.

Aluminium cooking utensils should not be used. The salts which come from these, though when taken in small quantities are not harmful, if taken over a long period become definitely so. Aluminium should be replaced with heavy quality enamel ware; or if this is not possible, the vegetables should be cooked in Patapar Papers (vegetable cooking parchment). If the Patapar Papers are used, the instructions given on the packet re the use of salt, soda, pepper, and butter etc. in the cooking process, should be disregarded.

Wholemeal flour and raw sugar are used exclusively in all the recipes in this book.

Use fine wholemeal flour. A little more liquid is needed than in cooking with white flour; but this must be added carefully, and only a little worked in at a time, as wholemeal is inclined to clog rather quickly, if care is not taken in mixing. It is quite easy to handle if properly mixed. Stickiness or crumbling in pastry, biscuits, scones, etc., is a sign that the quantities have not been correctly measured.

Raw sugar will mix easily and well if beaten properly. Sponges, etc., are light and fluffy if this is observed. They do not sink so readily as those made with white flour.

Puff, or flaky pastries are not so easily made with wholemeal as with white flour, but a rich short crust is easily made.

Cakes, biscuits, scones, etc., made with wholemeal flour are much fuller flavoured than those made with white; quite apart from the improved nutritive value.

A little water placed in the oven when it is turned on for baking cakes, and kept there during the cooking process, will keep them from getting too hard a crust and prevent them from burning. This does not apply to sponges.

Biscuits, or crisp cakes should not have the water placed in the oven.

Where coarse wheatmeal or oatmeal porridge has been recommended, take particular care with the cooking of this. The cooking process may need to be started at night, as some time is required to cook the coarse grains. Do not use any of the quickly-prepared, so-called "breakfast foods" on the market, as most of the goodness may have been extracted from them.

SWEETENING FRUIT

Avoid the use of sugar wherever possible for sweetening fruit. If the fruit is really ripe it should not need further sweetening. Honey is better than sugar for the purpose, but if either honey or sugar is to be added, put it in at the end of the cooking process.

Dried fruits for cooking should first be thoroughly washed, then soaked for 24 hours in water. Then cook them, at just below boiling point, in the same water in which they were soaked, until tender. They do not need long cooking, or any added sweetening, as dried fruits contain natural sugars.

Properly dried fruits are difficult to obtain. Commercially, it is easier to put fruits through a caustic and sulphuring preparation which tends to quicken the drying process and enhance the appearance of the fruit. Both processes have the effect of destroying food value. Fruits which have been subjected to no process other than drying in sun and air should be used whenever possible.

MEASUREMENT CONVERSION TABLE

¼ cup	=	60 mL	Breakfast cup	=	235 ml
⅓ cup	=	80 ml	1 gill (¼ pint)	=	140 ml
½ cup	=	125 ml	½ pint	=	285 ml
⅔ cup	=	160 ml	1 pint	=	570 ml
1 cup	=	250 ml	Quart	=	950 ml
Teacup	=	150 ml	Gallon	=	3800 ml
½ ounce	=	15 g	½ lb.	=	225 g
1 ounce	=	30 g	¾ lb.	=	340 g
¼ lb.	=	115 g	1 lb.	=	450 g

Low oven = 150°C = 300°F = Gas Mark 2
Mod. oven = 180°C = 360°F = Gas Mark 4
Hot oven = 220°C = 430°F = Gas Mark 7

Recipes Index

Soups 251
    Bran Stock 251
    Tomato Soup 251
    Celery Soup 251
    Parsnip Soup 251
    Spring soup 252
    Barley Broth 252
    Green Pea Soup 252
    Lentil Soup 252
    Brown Soup 253
    Curried Soup 253
    Lentil Puree 253
    Scotch Broth 253
    Asparagus Soup 254
    Bean Soup 254
    Vegetable Bouillon or Cleansing Soup 254
    Potato Soup 254
    Beetroot Soup 255
    Victoria Soup 255
    Cauliflower Soup 255
    Lettuce Soup 256
    Artichoke Soup 256
    Prize Tomato Soup 256
    Cabbage Soup 257
    Cream of Pumpkin Soup 257
    White Swiss Soup 257
    Almond Soup 258
    Vegetable Soup 258
    Mock Kidney Soup 258

 Cream of Celery 258

 Cream of Cucumber Soup 259

 Vegetable Marrow Soup 259

Gravies and Savoury Sauces 260

 Brown Gravy 260

 Wholemeal Gravy Sauce..260

 Tomato Sauce..260

 Onion Sauce 260

 Cream and Onion Sauce 260

 Cheese Sauce 261

 Tomato and Cheese Sauce – 1 261

 Tomato and Cheese Sauce – 2 261

 Celery, Tomato and Onion Sauce 261

 Mint Sauce 261

 Peas and Onion Sauce 262

Salads..263

 Everyday Salad 263

 Cabbage Salad 263

 Lettuce and Onion Salad 263

 Savoy and Leek Salad 263

 Apple and Carrot..263

 Mustard, Cress and Spinach 264

 Cucumber and Lettuce..264

 Lettuce and Green Peas 264

 New Potatoes and Spinach...264

 Watercress Salad 264

 Spinach and Carrot..264

 Potato and Celery 265

 Delicious Salad 265

 Watercress and Walnut 265

 Cauliflower and French Beans...265

Winter Salad	265
Banana and Nut	266
Date, Nut and Orange	266
Apple, Celery and Nut	266
Celery, Sprouts and Apple	266
Russian Salad	266

Unfired Savouries to Serve with Salads **267**

Egg	267
Nut – 1	267
Nut – 2	267
Cheese	267
Fruit Savoury Novelty (Not Unfired)	268

Salad Dressings **269**

Orange Cream	269
Almond Cream	269
Plain Mayonnaise That Will Keep	269
Special Mayonnaise Dressing	270
Plain Mayonnaise Dressing	270
Plain Dressings	270
French Fruit Dressing	271
Cream Salad Dressing	272

Hors d'Oeuvres **273**

Stuffed Tomato Hors d'Oeuvres	273
Lattice Hors d'Oeuvres	273
Prune Hors d'Oeuvres	273
Lettuce Rolls Hors d'Oeuvres	273
Bird's Nest Hors d'Oeuvres	273
Tip-Top Hors d'Oeuvres	274
Basket Hors d'Oeuvres	274
Vegetable and Egg Hors d'Oeuvres	274

 Grapefruit and Lettuce Hors d'Oeuvres 274
 Stuffed Prune Hors d'Oeuvres 275

Vegetable Dishes..276
 Stuffed Turnips..276
 Creamed Broad Beans 276
 Carrots Stewed In Butter 276
 Asparagus and Peas 276
 Creamed Peas and Carrots 277
 Stuffed Baked Tomatoes 277
 Marrow En Casserole 277
 Curried Marrow 277
 Cabbage Dutch..277
 Steamed Broad Bean Tops 278
 Baked Parsnip 278
 Creamed Cucumber 278
 Baked Onion and Cheese 278
 Carrot Au Gratin 279
 Baked Onion and Apple En Casserole...................................279
 Braised Lettuce..279
 Celery Au Gratin...279
 Baked Beetroot 280
 Beetroot In Butter..280
 Pumpkin Or Marrow In Butter..280
 Leeks Au Gratin 280
 Onion Rings...281
 Beetroot In Butter..281
 Stuffed Onions 281
 Savoury Marrow 281
 Creamed Sprouts 282

Savoury Vegetable and Meat Substitute Dishes........................283
 Savoury Mixed Grill...283

Haricot Dumplings	283
Nut Roast	283
Haricot Savoury	284
Risotto	284
Savoury Rice	284
Celery Pie	285
Cheese Cutlets	285
Almond Cutlets	286
Rice Loaf	286
Nut and Vegetable Rissoles	286
Nut Cutlets	286
Nut Croquettes	287
Stuffed Nut Roast	287
Rice Cheese Savoury	287
Summer Stew	288
Cauliflower, Tomato and Cheese Casserole	288
Nut and Vegetable Roast	288
Compote Vegetables and Forcemeat	289
Vegetable Roast	289
Summer Vegetables Medley	290
Nut Meat Supreme	290
Cauliflower and Nut Pie	291
Potatoes with Cheese	291
Cauliflower Roast	292
Potatoes Au Gratin	292
Onion Tart	292
Broad Bean Pie	293
Celery Loaf	293
Mushroom Cutlets	293
Macaroni and Nut Cutlets	294
Macaroni Cheese	294
Nut Meat	294

Cheese and Potato Roast 295
Dutch Pie 295
Granose Cheese Savoury 295
Granose Globes 295
Steamed Nut Savoury 296
Tokyo Savoury 296
Sicilian Savoury 296
Nut Meat Supreme 297
Savoury Rabbit* 297
Vegetable Savoury 298
Home-made Cheese 298
Nut Surprise 298
Vegetable Curry 299
Bean, Carrot and Peanut Loaf 299
Cabbage and Cheese Pie 299
Nut and Vegetable Pie 300
Cottage Cheese 300

Savoury Moulds and Jellies 301
Gelazone Galantine 301
Savoury Tomato Jelly 301
Cheese Mould 301
Lentil and Rice Mould 302
Savoury Jelly 302
Savoury Brawn 302

Egg Dishes, Soufflés, Omelettes, Savoury Batters, and Pancakes 303
Cheese Tart 303
Spinach Soufflé 303
Carrot Shape with Great Peas 303
Cheese and Tomato Soufflé 304
Onion Soufflé 304

Green Pea Soufflé 304
French Bean Soufflé 304
Cauliflower Soufflé 304
Swiss Eggs 305
Vegetable Soufflé 305
Spinach Entree 305
Eggs and Granose 305
Spinach Omelette 306
Walnut Omelette 306
Vegetable Omelette 306
Sylvan Eggs 306
Breadcrumb and Onion Omelette with Cheese Sauce 307
Fricassee of Eggs 307
Bombay Eggs 307
Curried Egg Rissoles 308
Egg Cutlets 308
Tomato Eggs 308
Baked Eggs 308
Egg and Potato Pie 309
Egg and Lentil Savoury 309
Savoury Batter (3 to 4 people) 309
Savoury Eggs 310

Fish Dishes 311
Savoury Fish Flan 311
Fish With Lemon Sauce 311
Fish Salad 311
Filleted Fish with Mushrooms 311
Fish Soufflé 312
Groper Rarebit 312
Fish Curry 312
Savoury Fish 313

Baked Fish 313
  Fish Savoury 313
  Fish Pie 314

Fruit Salads and Compotes 315
  Apple, Orange and Banana Salad 315
  Summer Fruit Salad 315
  Fig and Apple Salad 315
  Mixed Fruit Salad 315
  Spring Fruit Salad 315
  Winter Fruit Salad 316
  Winter Fruit Salad – 2 316
  Fruit Mousse 316
  Dried Fruit Salad 316
  Fruit Compote 317
  Fresh Fruit Compote 317
  Fruit Salad 317
  Peach Delicacy 317

Jellies, Trifles and Cold Sweets 318
  Date Dessert 318
  Fruit Moulds 318
  Almond Rice Mould 318
  Jelly Plum Pudding 318
  Rice Cream 319
  Apple Jelly 319
  Apple Delight 319
  Eden Pudding 320
  Peach Pudding 320
  Prune Whip 320
  Apricot and Boiled Custard 320
  Maple Walnut Sponge 321
  Blackberry Fool 321

Fruit Gelatine 321

Raisin Maple Blanc-Mange 321

Pineapple Junket 322

Moorish Pudding 322

Spanish Cream 322

Apple and Almond Cream 323

Baked, Boiled or Steamed Puddings, Tarts, Custards, etc. 324

Novelty Dried Fruit Pudding 324

Health Pudding 324

Date and Apple Charlotte 324

Short Crust 325

Plain Short Pastry 325

Rich Pastry 325

Plum Pudding 325

Apple Crisp 326

Raisin Rice 326

Apple Roll 326

Eve's Pudding 327

Fig Bran Pudding 327

Favourite Pudding 327

Prune Delicacy 328

Rhubarb Granose 328

Date Soufflé 328

Raisin Pudding 328

Date and Fig Pie with Chocolate Sauce 329

Cottage Pudding 329

Apple Goody 329

Prune, Apricot or Apple Betty 330

Prune Roll 330

Apple Puff 330

Carrot Pudding 330

Fig Pudding 331

Potato Pudding 331

Fig and Raisin Pudding 331

Prune and Fig Shape 331

Raisin or Sultana Pudding...332

Patricia Pudding 332

Steamed Date Pudding 332

Steamed Chocolate Pudding...332

Spanish Pudding...333

Steamed Treacle Sponge 333

Steamed Treacle Pudding 333

Stuffed Pears or Apples 333

Canary Pudding..334

Almond and Raisin Tart..334

Fig Roll 334

Sweet Wholemeal Pastry 335

Wholemeal Pastry — 1..335

Wholemeal Pastry — 2..335

Date or Fig Custard 335

Bananas in Lemon Syrup..336

Banana Flakes...336

Baked Bananas 336

Prune Meringue 336

Golden Custard..337

Fruit Sauces, etc. and Fillings for Tarts and Cakes 338

Lemon Curd 338

Swiss Jelly 338

Muscat Jelly 338

Banana Mincemeat 339

Fruit Sauce 339

Raisin Sauce..339

Lemon Sauce 339
Prune and Apple Sauce..339
Berry Sauce 340
Raw Berry Sauce 340
Honey Sauce 340
Orange Curd...340
Home Candied Peel..340
Fruit Filling — 1 341
Fruit Filling — 2 341
Fruit Filling — 3 341
Fruit Filling — 4 341
Raisin Cream Filling..341
Raisin Caramel Frosting 342

Wholemeal Breads, Scones, Loaves, Slices.........................343
Treacle Bread 343
Wholemeal Bread..343
Excellent Wholemeal Bread 343
Family Wholemeal Bread 344
Wholemeal Scones..344
Potato Scones...344
Pumpkin Scones..345
Bran Scones...345
Spice Scones..345
Wholemeal Fruit Loaf 345
Raisin Scones..346
Love Knots...346
Oatmeal Slices 346
Muscatel Bread..346
Wholemeal Honey Scones...347
Wholemeal Nut Loaf...347
Nut and Date Loaf..347

Bran Muffins 347
Currant Bread 348
Oatcakes 348
Rusks 348

Biscuits: Plain, Savoury and Sweet 349
Rolled Oat Biscuits 349
Plain Wholemeal Biscuits 349
Savoury Cheese Biscuits 349
Wholemeal Cheese Straws 349
Cheese and Potato Biscuits 350
Lunchies 350
Nut Biscuits 350
Fruit Biscuits 350
Three-A-Penny Biscuits 351
Lemon Rings 351
Sponge Biscuits 351
Golden Syrup Biscuits 351
Butter Biscuits 352
Honey Biscuits 352
Lunch Squares 352
Date Crackers 353
Bran Biscuits 353

Fruit, Sponge, and Small Cakes 354
Sultana Lunch Cake 354
Ginger Bran Cake 354
Peace Cake 354
Bran Parkins 355
Wholemeal Walnut Cake 355
Nut Cake 355
Caramel Cake 356
Topsy Turvy Cake 356

Economical Wholemeal Cake	356
Short Cake	357
Orange Cake	357
Coconut Meringue Shortcake	357
Wholemeal Cake (No Eggs)	357
Iced Wholemeal Cake	358
Sponge Cake	358
Bran Cake De Luxe	358
Chester Cake	359
Nutties	359
Fruit Snaps	359
Walnut Brownies	360
Walnut Crisps	360
Date Caramel Cake	360
Chocolate Afghans	360
Lemon Drop Cookies	361
Crunchies	361
Choice Christmas Cake	361
Light Wholemeal Cake	362
Lunch Rock Buns	362
Shortcake	362
Almond Macaroons	362
Raisin Munchers	363
Date Surprises	363
Wigmore Cake	363
Prune Cake	364
Good Fruit Cake	364
Madeira Cake	364
Plain Wholemeal Raisin Cake	364
Wholemeal Sponge Cake	365
Honey Short Cake	365
Rolled Oats Shortbread	365

Peanut Cookies 366
　Wholemeal Fruit Cake 366
　Trilby Cakes 366
　Cheese Cakes 367

Sandwiches **368**
　Pastes For Sandwich Fillings 368
　Plain Bread and Butter Sandwiches 368
　Biscuit Sandwiches 369
　Cheese Sandwiches (Various) 369

Beverages **370**
　Welsh Nectar 370
　Cereal Drinks 370
　Lemon Delight 371
　Grapefruit and Apricot 371

Soups

BRAN STOCK

INGREDIENTS.—A handful of bran to 2 pints of water or vegetable stock.

METHOD.—Simmer gently 2 hours; then strain. Use as a base for soups or for moistening savouries. This stock abounds in mineral salts.

TOMATO SOUP

INGREDIENTS.—1 pint bran or vegetable stock, 2 large onions, 1 breakfast cup of milk, 2 tablespoons brown sago, 2 lbs. skinned tomatoes.

METHOD.—Simmer 1 hour without milk. Strain, add milk and parsley. Serve at once.

CELERY SOUP

INGREDIENTS.—1 quart bran or vegetable stock. Coarse outside lettuce leaves, chopped celery, teaspoon celery salt, wholemeal flour to thicken.

METHOD.—Simmer 1½ hours, put through sieve and thicken.

PARSNIP SOUP

INGREDIENTS.—2 lb. parsnips, 1 large grated carrot, 3 onions, 1 quart bran or vegetable stock.

METHOD.—Cut parsnips and onions small, add carrot. Simmer 2 hours and rub through sieve. Add 1 tablespoon chopped mint just before serving.

SPRING SOUP

INGREDIENTS. — ½ pint stock, ½ pint milk, 1 lb. spinach, 1 lb. coarse lettuce, ½ lb. young dandelion leaves, a few sorrel leaves, 2 or 3 bay leaves if obtainable, 1 ounce butter, 2 egg yolks.

METHOD. — Cook leaves gently in stock till tender. Add milk and butter, and heat. Beat eggs in bowl in which soup is to be served, adding a little warm soup, then gradually add the remainder of the hot soup (the leaves to be strained from the stock).

BARLEY BROTH

INGREDIENTS. — 1 teacup unpolished barley, 1 large bunch leeks, 1 large grated carrot, 2 bay leaves if obtainable, I dessertspoonful of vegetable or olive oil.

METHOD. — Simmer all for 2 hours, adding the oil 10 minutes before serving.

GREEN PEA SOUP

INGREDIENTS. — 1 breakfast cup dried green peas soaked overnight, ½ cabbage, 3 onions, 2 tablespoons seedless raisins, sprig of mint, 1 quart stock.

METHOD. — Chop cabbage, onions and raisins fine. Simmer all for 2 hours and rub through sieve.

LENTIL SOUP

INGREDIENTS. — ½ lb. lentils, 2 ounces brown rice, 3 quarts stock, ½ teaspoon celery salt, 2 large turnips, 2 carrots, 2 onions, thyme, 1 teaspoon Marmite.

METHOD. — Grate all vegetables and simmer with lentils and rice for 2 hours. Add Marmite just before serving.

BROWN SOUP

INGREDIENTS. — ½ packet soaked butter beans, 1 swede, 1 onion, 2 carrots, ½ lb. spinach. Few celery tops and outside stalks, ½ teaspoon herbs, 1 quart stock.

METHOD. — Simmer all together for 3 hours, rub through sieve.

CURRIED SOUP

INGREDIENTS. — 1 lb. potatoes, ½ lb. each carrots, onions, sweet apples, ¼ lb. seedless raisins, 1 tablespoon brown sago, ½ teaspoon cinnamon, 1 level tablespoon curry powder, rather less than 2 pints stock.

METHOD. — Chop vegetables, raisins and apples and simmer all ingredients 3 hours. Rub through sieve.

LENTIL PUREE

INGREDIENTS. — 1 lb. lentils, 1 sliced onion, few cloves, 1 teaspoon mixed herbs, ½ teaspoon celery salt, 1 tablespoon chopped parsley, 1 ounce butter.

METHOD. — Cook all except butter and parsley in 1 quart of water until mushed. Put through a sieve. Cream butter and add, then add parsley. Serve hot with dry toast or cheese biscuits.

SCOTCH BROTH

INGREDIENTS. — 1 large carrot, 1 leek, 1 onion, ½ cauliflower, ¼ large turnip, 1 or 2 celery stalks, spinach, a few green cabbage leaves, 1 lb. fresh peas or ½ lb. dried ones soaked overnight.

METHOD. — Wash vegetables and chop. Melt 1 ounce butter and add onion, brown, and add 2 quarts water and vegetables. Cook gently 2 hours.

ASPARAGUS SOUP

INGREDIENTS and METHOD.—One large bunch of asparagus. Place in 1 pint slightly salted water and cook until soft. Rub through sieve. Reheat with about ½ pint milk, taking care that milk does not quite boil. Add a little butter.

BEAN SOUP

INGREDIENTS.—2 cups lima or haricot beans soaked overnight, 1 large onion, 1 green pepper, 1 clove garlic, large piece butter, juice of 1 lemon.

METHOD.—Add 2 quarts of water and more as becomes necessary, and cook slowly 2 to 4 hours.

VEGETABLE BOUILLON OR CLEANSING SOUP

INGREDIENTS.—Spinach, carrots, turnips, parsnips, sprouts, onions, etc.

METHOD.—Grate and put into a large saucepan and well cover with water. Simmer 2 or 3 hours. A little Marmite may be added just before serving and after the soup has been strained. Excellent to take during a fast.

POTATO SOUP

INGREDIENTS.—2 lb. potatoes, 2 onions, ½ pint water, ½ pint milk, 2 ounces butter, salt to taste, 1 tablespoon chopped parsley, 1 ounce grated cheese.

METHOD.—Grate potatoes and onions and boil gently with water. Add milk but do not boil. Five minutes before serving add butter, cheese and parsley.

BEETROOT SOUP

INGREDIENTS.—1 lb. beetroot, 1 large carrot, 1 large onion, 1 lemon, parsley, cream.

METHOD.—Put 2 ounces butter and onion in covered pan. Grate beetroot and carrot and add to onion with 1½ pints water. Simmer 1½ hours. Then add teaspoon Marmite, juice of lemon, salt, and pinch of sugar, parsley. Thicken with a dessertspoon wholemeal flour and a beaten egg. Serve with fresh cream.

VICTORIA SOUP

INGREDIENTS.—1 cupful each of grated onion and carrot, ½ cupful celery, 2 tablespoons butter, 2 teaspoons flour, 2 quarts water.

METHOD.—Brown the chopped vegetables in butter; then add boiling water. Cook till tender, then thicken with the wholemeal flour.

CAULIFLOWER SOUP

INGREDIENTS.—1 cauliflower, 2 sticks celery, 1 onion, 2 ounces butter, 2 ounces wholemeal flour.

METHOD.—Cut cauliflower in quarters and after soaking in slightly salted water, boil for 10 minutes; add chopped onion and chopped celery and cook till tender. Strain, saving water. Reserve a few flowerets and rub the rest of the vegetables through a sieve. Melt butter and stir in flour. Add ½ pint milk and 1½ pints water in which vegetables were cooked. Stir till boiling. Add puree and simmer 10 minutes. Put flowerets in a well heated tureen and pour soup over them.

LETTUCE SOUP

INGREDIENTS.—lettuce, 1 quart stock (1 pint milk and 1 pint water), 2 tablespoons wholemeal flour, 2 tablespoons butter, 2 tablespoons lemon juice.

METHOD.—Melt butter and add flour, add half hot stock and bring to boil and season. Cook lettuce in other half stock and rub through sieve when tender. Mix well with other sauce, beat well; add lemon juice and serve very hot.

ARTICHOKE SOUP

INGREDIENTS.—1 lb. artichokes, 1 large onion, 1 gill (140 ml) cream, 1 pint milk.

METHOD.—Wash artichokes and rub skin with a cloth and a little salt. Steam till tender. Chop onion and stew in a little milk. Add to the artichokes and put through sieve. Reheat with milk and cream. Thicken slightly with wholemeal flour if necessary.

PRIZE TOMATO SOUP

INGREDIENTS.—Green leaves of cabbage, stick of celery, 1 grated swede turnip, 1 grated carrot, 1 grated unpeeled potato, 1 large onion, ½ lb. tomatoes, 1 gill (140 ml) peas and beans, sprig of thyme, 1 bay leaf, 1 tablespoon each of lentils and unpolished barley.

METHOD.—Soak peas and beans overnight, cut cabbage and celery and cook slowly 1½ hours. Strain. Fry onions and tomatoes in butter 15 minutes and add to cabbage and celery stock, together with the potato, carrot, turnip, peas, beans, lentils and barley. Simmer slowly 1½ hours and then add 1 gill (140 ml) of milk and 1 dessertspoon of Marmite.

CABBAGE SOUP

INGREDIENTS.—2 cabbages, 1½ pints water, 1 pint milk, 1 onion, 1 ounce butter, 2 ounces brown sago, parsley, a little salt and pepper.

METHOD.—Shred cabbage finely and soak in salted water half hour. Gently stew the onion and butter and parsley 5 minutes. Add cabbage and stir well. Add the water and simmer 15 minutes. Stir in sago; cook 10 minutes. Add milk and bring to just below Boiling point.

CREAM OF PUMPKIN SOUP

INGREDIENTS.—1 lb. pumpkin, 1 tablespoon of butter, ½ pint of boiling water, 1½ pints of milk, 2 tablespoons of flour.

METHOD.—Peel pumpkin and cut into slices. Put into a saucepan with water and cook until mashed. Rub through a sieve and add the milk, butter and flour, rubbing the flour smooth with a little milk. Reheat, season to taste, serve very hot.

(Cream of carrot or parsnip may be made the same way.)

WHITE SWISS SOUP

INGREDIENTS.—½ cup of brown rice, 1½ cups of milk, a little wholemeal flour, 1 small onion, 1 egg yolk, 2 cups of water, 1 potato.

METHOD.—Boil rice in water and add onion and potato; when these are cooked add milk and bring to just below boiling point. Beat well the egg yolk and the flour (about a teaspoonful) and stir into the soup. Season to taste, rub through sieve, reheat and serve.

ALMOND SOUP

INGREDIENTS. — 2 ounces ground almonds, 1 onion, 1½ pints stock, 1 pint milk, 3 or 4 young carrots, 1 gill (140 ml) cream.

METHOD. — Cook onions in butter; add carrots cut up and cook a few minutes. Add hot stock and simmer 1 hour. Rub through a sieve, add the ground almonds and just before serving, the milk and cream.

VEGETABLE SOUP

INGREDIENTS. — 3 each carrots, potatoes, onions, turnips, 2 parsnips, celery stalks, 3 pints milk, a good-sized piece of butter, chopped parsley.

METHOD. — Bring chopped vegetables to boil in water, cook till tender and rub through a coarse sieve, to make in all about 3 pints. Add the 3 pints of milk and butter and reheat. Sprinkle with parsley before serving.

MOCK KIDNEY SOUP

INGREDIENTS and METHOD. — Soak 1 lb. lentils overnight in plenty of water. Cut up any available vegetables such as carrot, turnip, onion, celery, etc., and fry them in butter until brown. Add 1 cup of brown breadcrumbs. Pour all into the steeped lentils and bring to the boil. Then simmer till tender. Force through sieve with a wooden spoon. If possible add pieces of chopped mushroom fried in a little butter.

CREAM OF CELERY

INGREDIENTS. — 2 cups of diced celery, 3 tablespoons of butter, 4 cups of milk, 4 tablespoons wholemeal flour, 4 cups cold water.

METHOD. — Cook celery in water till tender, rub butter and flour together. Add half of this to water left on celery when done. Heat milk and add remaining flour and butter, combine with celery, etc., and season to taste.

CREAM OF CUCUMBER SOUP

INGREDIENTS. — 2 cups of milk, 1 cup of water, not stock, 1½ cups of diced cucumber, 1 onion, grated, 2 tablespoons of flour, salt.

METHOD. — Put the cucumber on to cook in the water. Add the grated onion and milk and bring to boil. Then blend flour with a little milk and stir in. Add a fair-sized piece of butter and cook very gently for 5 minutes.

VEGETABLE MARROW SOUP

INGREDIENTS. — 1 lb. vegetable marrow, 1½ pints stock, 1 onion, 1 ounce butter, 1 ounce flour, ½ pint milk.

METHOD. — Peel and slice marrow and use 1 lb. to 1 quart soup. Simmer gently with onion for half hour and put through a sieve. Mix flour smoothly with milk and butter and add to the marrow puree. Reheat and sprinkle with parsley before serving.

Gravies and Savoury Sauces

BROWN GRAVY

INGREDIENTS.—2 ounces browned wholemeal flour, 2 ounces butter, 1 onion, ¾ pint stock or water, a little Marmite.

METHOD.—Brown butter in pan, add and cook onions until quite brown, add browned flour, stirring gently, then stock. Cook well and keep well stirred. Season and strain.

WHOLEMEAL GRAVY SAUCE

INGREDIENTS and METHOD.—Half pint strong vegetable stock. Two tablespoons wholemeal flour; seasoning. Cook 5 minutes.

TOMATO SAUCE

INGREDIENTS and METHOD.—Cut up tomatoes to make 1 pint. Cook with very finely chopped onion about 10 minutes. Add 1 tablespoon flour blended with same amount of butter; allow to boil for a few minutes. A little salt if desired. May be strained if liked.

ONION SAUCE

INGREDIENTS and METHOD.—Slice onions and brown them in butter. Add a little flour and enough stock or milk to make the right consistency. Cook and season.

CREAM AND ONION SAUCE

INGREDIENTS and METHOD.—Cook 1 cup of grated onion in a little water. Blend 2 tablespoons melted butter with 2 of flour. Add to onions, stirring well, and add ½ cup of cream or milk.

CHEESE SAUCE

INGREDIENTS. — Half pint vegetable stock, 2 tablespoons wholemeal flour, 3 ounces grated cheese.

METHOD. — Blend and cook stock and flour for a few minutes; add grated cheese. Milk may be substituted for the vegetable stock.

TOMATO AND CHEESE SAUCE — 1

INGREDIENTS and METHOD. — Cook 1 cup of grated onion in a little water. Blend 2 tablespoons each of butter and flour; add 1 cup tomato to the cooked onion, then the butter and flour. Cook together for a few minutes. Season and add a little cream or milk before serving.

TOMATO AND CHEESE SAUCE — 2

INGREDIENTS and METHOD. — Mash ¼ lb. cheese to a paste with a little milk or water. Add 1 cup of hot tomato sauce and mix well. Reheat before serving.

CELERY, TOMATO AND ONION SAUCE

INGREDIENTS and METHOD. — Cook half an onion, 1 cup celery and 1 cup tomatoes in water till tender, then mash through colander. Blend 1 tablespoon butter with 1 table-spoon wholemeal flour. Mix with other ingredients and stir together for a few minutes till cooked.

MINT SAUCE

INGREDIENTS and METHOD. — One cup finely chopped mint, ¼ cup raw sugar, ½ cup lemon juice. Stand 1 hour, warm, but do not boil.

PEAS AND ONION SAUCE

INGREDIENTS and METHOD.—Simmer 2 finely chopped onions in a little water. When tender add ½ cupful cooked peas and 2 diced tomatoes. Season with a little celery salt and butter.

Salads

EVERYDAY SALAD

INGREDIENTS and METHOD.—Finely grated raw vegetables in any combination with either lettuce, spinach, dandelion leaves, silver-beet leaves, turnip tops, etc., for the green element. For example: An excellent and inexpensive salad may be made of grated carrot, turnip, beetroot, apple, a few raisins, and heart of white cabbage.

CABBAGE SALAD

INGREDIENTS and METHOD.—One small heart of cabbage, small heart celery, 2 tomatoes. Cut up cabbage and celery finely, skin and quarter tomatoes. (Diced apple may replace tomato.)

LETTUCE AND ONION SALAD

METHOD.—Shred lettuce and chop onion finely. Mix well together and sprinkle with grated cheese.

SAVOY AND LEEK SALAD

INGREDIENTS and METHOD.—One heart of savoy, 1 leek, 1 parsnip, a few dandelion leaves. Scrape and grate parsnip, thinly shred leeks, savoy and dandelion leaves. Mix together.

APPLE AND CARROT

METHOD.—Grate the carrot and chop the apple. Sprinkle with grated nut.

MUSTARD, CRESS AND SPINACH

METHOD.—Chop all, mix well, and serve with either grated cheese or nuts.

CUCUMBER AND LETTUCE

INGREDIENTS and METHOD.—One good sized lettuce, cucumber. Wash and arrange lettuce on dish. Dice unpeeled cucumber and place among lettuce leaves. Dress with lemon juice and olive oil.

LETTUCE AND GREEN PEAS

METHOD.—Use lettuce leaves as cups and fill with green peas, cooked or raw, sprinkled with finely chopped mint and dressed with cream dressing.

NEW POTATOES AND SPINACH

METHOD.—Cook and dice potatoes. Chop up spinach and mix well. Serve with curd cheese.

WATERCRESS SALAD

INGREDIENTS and METHOD.—Watercress, hard boiled eggs. Wash and chop watercress; cut garlic into very tiny pieces; mix well and put sliced egg on top.

SPINACH AND CARROT

INGREDIENTS and METHOD.—Quantity of perpetual spinach, grated carrot, 1 level teaspoon chopped garlic. Mix well and serve with grated cheese.

POTATO AND CELERY

INGREDIENTS and METHOD.—Two heads celery, 2 steamed cold potatoes. Dice and dress with lemon juice and oil.

DELICIOUS SALAD

INGREDIENTS and METHOD.—Mix grated raw cauliflower, apple, celeriac or chopped celery, and heap on lettuce. Add a sprinkling of seeded raisins and decorate with slices of hard boiled egg or thinly sliced cheese.

WATERCRESS AND WALNUT

INGREDIENTS.—Watercress, radishes, carrot, cucumber, walnuts.
METHOD.—Make a centre of grated raw carrots and arrange cress round it. Decorate with chopped radishes and cubes of unpeeled cucumber. Sprinkle with walnuts.

CAULIFLOWER AND FRENCH BEANS

METHOD.—Line a bowl with lettuce leaves and pile sprigs of cold cooked cauliflower in centre. Make a dressing of 6 tablespoons of olive oil, 1 tablespoon lemon juice, and a little chopped parsley, and pour half of this over the cauliflower. Beat up the yolk of an egg and add rest of dressing gradually to it. Toss cold cooked beans in this and arrange round cauliflower. Sprinkle with parsley and serve.

WINTER SALAD

INGREDIENTS and METHOD.—Grated carrots, parsnips, turnips, a little horseradish, shredded cabbage, or Brussels sprouts and chopped onion. Mix.

BANANA AND NUT

METHOD.—Slice a banana very thinly and mix with 2 tablespoons chopped nuts and 1 tablespoon salad dressing. Serve with lettuce or watercress on bed of cooked rice.

DATE, NUT AND ORANGE

METHOD.—Mix stoned chopped dates with chopped nuts and blend with an orange cut into bits. Serve on lettuce leaves and dress with oil.

APPLE, CELERY AND NUT

METHOD.—Chop apple and celery finely and bind with cream salad dressing. Sprinkle generously with chopped nuts and serve with lettuce or watercress.

CELERY, SPROUTS AND APPLE

METHOD.—Chop celery into ½-inch pieces. Mix in about half the quantity of finely shredded sprouts and of grated apple. Arrange on lettuce leaves and sprinkle with 2 tablespoons nut oil.

RUSSIAN SALAD

INGREDIENTS and METHOD.—Lettuce shredded finely. A mixture of any and every kind of cooked vegetable, e.g. peas, beans, beetroot, carrot, turnip, asparagus, potato, tomato. Dress with cream dressing.

Unfired Savouries to Serve with Salads

EGG

INGREDIENTS and METHOD.—2 cups finely chopped cabbage or sea kale. 1 dessertspoon finely chopped mint. tablespoon melted butter, in which has been dissolved 1 scant teaspoon Marmite. Add beaten egg to butter and Marmite; stir in cabbage and mint; shape, and roll in Corn flakes.

NUT—1

INGREDIENTS.—2 cups raw, finely chopped cabbage, 2 ounces milled nuts, 1 tablespoon finely grated onion, 1 teaspoon savoury herbs, 2 tablespoons grated raw swede.

METHOD.—Mix these ingredients with vegetable stock, flavoured with Marmite. Shape and roll in dextrinised wholemeal bread crumbs.

NUT—2

INGREDIENTS.—½ teacup milled nuts, 1 teacup crushed Corn flakes, 1 teaspoon celery salt, 1 teacup finely minced onions, 1 tablespoon raw cucumber juice or pulp.

METHOD.—Mix and shape into little balls; roll in milled nuts.

CHEESE

INGREDIENTS.—1 cup mashed potatoes, 2 ounces grated cheese, little melted butter, 1 cup grated raw beetroot, ½ cup finely diced celery.

METHOD.—Mix together, and roll in finely grated cheese.

FRUIT SAVOURY NOVELTY (Not Unfired)

INGREDIENTS.—12 ounces wholemeal flour, 6 ounces grated cheese, 3 bananas, ½ teaspoon cinnamon, 4 ounces butter, 6 ounces seeded raisins, 1 dessertspoon gelatine, 1½ pints boiling water.

METHOD.—Soak raisins over night in the water; strain and make quantity of liquid up to 1 pint. Sprinkle in cinnamon, and stir in gelatine which has been previously mixed in a little of the cold water. Heat, but do not boil. Pour this over raisins and sliced bananas. Set. Make a paste of butter, flour and cheese mixed with a little water. Roll lightly and line patty pans. Fill with fruit mixture, cover with pastry, and bake 15 minutes in moderate oven.

Salad Dressings

ORANGE CREAM

INGREDIENTS.—About 2 ounces cottage cheese, 1 level dessertspoon honey, 2 ounces ground sweet almonds, juice 1½ large oranges.

METHOD.—Thoroughly mix honey and cheese; add very gradually the orange juice till all is smooth and creamy. Stir in ground almonds last.

ALMOND CREAM

INGREDIENTS.—About 2 ounces cottage cheese, 1 ounce ground almonds, 1 tablespoon cream, 2 tablespoons raw carrot juice.

METHOD.—Make carrot juice by grating and squeezing pulp in muslin bag. Mix cheese, almonds and cream lightly together, adding carrot juice gradually.

PLAIN MAYONNAISE THAT WILL KEEP

INGREDIENTS.—3 tablespoons wholemeal flour, fine, 2 tablespoons butter, 2 egg yolks, 1 teaspoon salt, a little pepper, 1 cup olive oil, 1½ to 2 cups lukewarm water, juice of one or two lemons, according to taste, about a dessertspoon made mustard.

METHOD.—Melt butter, add flour, mix well, add luke warm water, stirring till thick over a slow heat. Remove from fire and add lemon juice. Put egg yolks and seasonings into a basin, beat well. Add this to flour and butter, beating continuously. Add gradually olive oil, about o f a cup at a time, and beat thoroughly. Will keep a long time.

SPECIAL MAYONNAISE DRESSING

INGREDIENTS.—1 cup of whipped cream, juice of 1 lemon, 1 teaspoon honey, 3 tablespoons vegetable oil.

METHOD.—Beat the oil, honey and lemon juice till thoroughly mixed. Slowly add whipped cream. This will keep in covered jar.

PLAIN MAYONNAISE DRESSING

INGREDIENTS.—1 yolk of egg, 1 gill (140 ml) salad oil, 1 tablespoon lemon juice, pinch salt.

METHOD.—Stir the yolk of egg with the salt and add oil drop by drop. As it begins to thicken beat well and add oil in larger quantities. Add lemon juice carefully last of all.

PLAIN DRESSINGS

No. 1—

INGREDIENTS and METHOD.—3 spoonfuls of lemon juice to 5 of oil. Add gradually, stirring all the time.

No. 2—

INGREDIENTS.—2 eggs, 4 tablespoons cream, 3 tablespoons lemon juice, ½ teaspoon celery salt, a little mustard if desired, a little grated onion.

METHOD.—Beat yolks well, add onion, then cream, lemon juice, celery salt, and mustard. Beat all thoroughly.

No. 3—

INGREDIENTS and METHOD.—Mix 1 teaspoon mustard, ½ teaspoon celery salt, 1 teaspoon chopped garlic, 1½ dessertspoons olive or nut oil. Beat all thoroughly together.

No. 4 —

INGREDIENTS and METHOD. — 1 teacup rich milk, 1 well beaten egg yolk, 2 tablespoons lemon juice, a little mustard and ½ teaspoon celery salt if liked. Mix and beat well.

No. 5 —

INGREDIENTS and METHOD. — Mix till creamy 1 cup raw sugar and 2 tablespoons butter. Add unbeaten white of an egg a little at a time, stir for 10 minutes, then add juice of half lemon.

No. 6 —

INGREDIENTS and METHOD. — 2 tablespoons raw sugar to 1 cup of sour milk. Add lemon juice to taste and mix well.

No. 7 —

INGREDIENTS and METHOD. — Beat very lightly 2 egg yolks, add ½ cup thin honey, juice ½ lemon, pinch salt. Cook in double saucepan, stirring all the time till mixture thickens. Cool slightly and fold in stiffly beaten egg whites.

No. 8 —

INGREDIENTS and METHOD. — Cook together 3 tablespoons finely chopped onion, the same of finely chopped celery, and 1 cup of tomato sauce, till soft. Rub through coarse sieve.

FRENCH FRUIT DRESSING

INGREDIENTS and METHOD. — Mix with egg beater the following: 4 tablespoons olive oil, 3 tablespoons orange juice, 3 tablespoons lemon juice, 1 tablespoon honey.

CREAM SALAD DRESSING

INGREDIENTS. — 3 tablespoons olive oil, 2½ tablespoons lemon juice, 3 tablespoons cream, 1 tablespoon chopped parsley, onion, chives, tarragon, ½ teaspoon salt.

METHOD. — Beat yolks well, add onion, then cream, lemon juice, celery salt, and mustard. Beat all thoroughly.

Hors d'Oeuvres

STUFFED TOMATO HORS D'OEUVRES

METHOD.—Cut a thin slice from the top of each tomato. Scoop out centre carefully. Chop cucumber and season with a little onion and mix with pulp. Fill tomato cases with this mixture. Pour over French dressing and serve on large lettuce leaf. Substitute finely diced celery for cucumber.

LATTICE HORS D'OEUVRES

METHOD.—Some flat pieces of lettuce leaf. Cut strips of cucumber and put in lattice design on lettuce leaf. Surround with ring of grated carrot. Put a little grated beetroot in centre of cucumber and place a blanched almond on top.

PRUNE HORS D'OEUVRES

METHOD.—Remove stone and fill cavity with mixture of chopped cucumber, chopped apple and cream cheese. Serve on lettuce leaf.

LETTUCE ROLLS HORS D'OEUVRES

METHOD.—Spread a crisp piece of lettuce with cream cheese, roll up and tie with nasturtium leaf.

BIRD'S NEST HORS D'OEUVRES

METHOD.—Allow 1 slice cooked beetroot per person and on it arrange a nest of mustard and cress. Drop in "eggs" of cream cheese dipped in milled nuts.

TIP-TOP HORS D'OEUVRES

INGREDIENTS and METHOD.—Tomatoes, asparagus, lettuce, a little sour cream. Slice tomatoes about ½-inch thick, cut out small rounds from centre of each and insert 4 or 5 asparagus tips. Serve with sour cream dotted round lettuce.

BASKET HORS D'OEUVRES

INGREDIENTS and METHOD.—Hard boiled eggs, chopped parsley, mustard and cress, olives. Cut eggs lengthwise, mix yolk with chopped parsley, replace and put a slice of stuffed olive in centre. Select a piece of cress stalk to form handle, surround with mustard and cress.

VEGETABLE AND EGG HORS D'OEUVRES

INGREDIENTS and METHOD.—One large carrot, 1 large potato, green peas. Steam all. Raw beetroot, celery and tomato. Hard boiled eggs. Dice carrot and potato and mix in peas, pour over this a mayonnaise. Shred the beetroot and soak in lemon juice a little while, slice tomato and chop celery. Halve eggs and lightly cover with mayonnaise. Serve on individual dishes with lettuce leaf foundation, arranging the ingredients in little heaps.

GRAPEFRUIT AND LETTUCE HORS D'OEUVRES

METHOD.—Peel grapefruit and peel each section without breaking. Arrange about 6 sections on a lettuce leaf. Lightly sprinkle with shredded carrot, mix a little olive oil and lemon juice and pour 1 teaspoon over each helping before serving.

STUFFED PRUNE HORS D'OEUVRES

METHOD.—Soak some prunes in lemon juice until swollen and soft. Remove stones and fill with cream cheese and chopped nuts. Surround prunes with sliced tomato and cucumber on lettuce leaf.

Vegetable Dishes

STUFFED TURNIPS

INGREDIENTS and METHOD.—6 large turnips. Scoop out centres and peel, leaving ½-inch cup. Simmer till tender and strain. To ½ lb. chopped onion add 2 teaspoons chopped sage and some turnip centres. Cook these in 1 gill (140 ml) of milk 20 minutes. Add 3 ounces brown breadcrumbs. Stuff turnips with this mixture and grate over butter and cheese. Brown in oven for 15 minutes.

CREAMED BROAD BEANS

INGREDIENTS.—To 2 pints broad beans allow ½ pint vegetable stock, 1 egg yolk, 1 gill (140 ml) cream, mint, parsley.

METHOD.—Partly cook beans and put into casserole dish with stock and seasoning. Simmer till stock is reduced, add yolk and cream, reheat and serve at once.

CARROTS STEWED IN BUTTER

INGREDIENTS.—2 lb. carrots, 1 chopped onion, juice of ½ lemon, 3 tablespoons flour.

METHOD.—Cut carrots into rounds and stew with butter and onion. Add lemon juice, simmer for 40 minutes. Add thickening of wholemeal flour and chopped parsley.

ASPARAGUS AND PEAS

METHOD.—Cook equal quantities of asparagus and peas together, the asparagus cut into ½-inch pieces. Serve with butter sauce.

CREAMED PEAS AND CARROTS

METHOD. — Cook equal parts of cubed carrots and peas in as small amount of water as possible till tender, cover with milk and thicken with butter and wholemeal flour.

STUFFED BAKED TOMATOES

METHOD. — Cut slice off top of tomatoes, scoop out centre and fill with mixture of wholemeal breadcrumbs, cheese and chopped parsley. Replace tops and bake in moderate oven.

MARROW EN CASSEROLE

METHOD. — Prepare tender young marrow. Put thinly sliced onion in bottom of a casserole dish; then marrow cut in two. Cover with slices of blanched tomatoes. Mix dessertspoon flour with tablespoon butter and dot in little balls over marrow. Cover closely and simmer till tender. May be served on dry toast as a savoury.

CURRIED MARROW

METHOD. — Slice a large onion; add marrow cut into cubes. Sprinkle over 1 dessertspoon wholemeal flour, 1 teaspoon curry powder, 1 tablespoon butter. Simmer till tender.

CABBAGE DUTCH

INGREDIENTS and METHOD. — Cut up finely equal quantities of cabbage and unpeeled apples. Add half as much chopped onion as cabbage. Cook with very little water in a closely covered saucepan. Stir frequently. Cook 1 to 1½ hours over slow heat. When half done add 1 tablespoon butter.

STEAMED BROAD BEAN TOPS

METHOD. — Wash and steam without adding any water for half-hour. Chop with a little butter.

BAKED PARSNIP

METHOD. — Split parsnips in two and boil in small amount of water until tender. Place in baking dish, add a piece of butter and any water that may be left. Brown lightly, basting 2 or 3 times.

CREAMED CUCUMBER

INGREDIENTS. — 2 lbs. cucumber, ½ pint wholemeal sauce, 1 chopped onion, 1 tablespoon wholemeal flour, 1 grated carrot, teaspoon chopped parsley, 2 ounces butter, 1 gill (140 ml) water, a little milk, 1 gill cream.

METHOD. — Cut cucumber into ½-inch slices and simmer 10 to 15 minutes. Sauce: Stew chopped onion, carrot and parsley in butter. Add 1 gill (140 ml) of water in which cucumber was cooked; mix flour with milk, add and simmer 5 Minutes. Add the cream, mix in strained cucumber, and serve sprinkled with parsley.

BAKED ONION AND CHEESE

INGREDIENTS. — 4 large onions, 4 ounces cheese, wholemeal breadcrumbs.

METHOD. — Partly steam onions and chop them roughly and put into well buttered dish with a very little vegetable stock. Season and cover with an equal mixture of breadcrumbs and cheese. Bake until nicely browned.

CARROT AU GRATIN

INGREDIENTS.—1½ lb. grated carrot, 5 ounces cheese, 1 ounce butter, wholemeal bread crumbs.

METHOD.—Steam carrots and mash; add butter and grated cheese. Put in buttered pie-dish, cover with breadcrumbs and bake until lightly brown.

BAKED ONION AND APPLE EN CASSEROLE

INGREDIENTS.—4 medium-sized apples, 6 onions, ⅔ cup of water, 1 tablespoon butter.

METHOD.—Slice onions thinly. Peel, core and slice apples. Arrange in buttered casserole dish, add water, dot butter over and bake in moderate oven with lid on for 30 minutes. Remove cover and brown about another fifteen minute

BRAISED LETTUCE

INGREDIENTS.—6 cabbage lettuce, 1 onion, 1 tablespoon cream, 1 tablespoon chopped herbs, 1 tablespoon wholemeal flour.

METHOD.—Shred lettuce, chop onion and brown in butter; add lettuce, sprinkle in flour and stew gently for 20 minutes. Before serving add herbs and cream.

CELERY AU GRATIN

INGREDIENTS.—3 large heads of celery, 8 ounces grated cheese, milk, wholemeal breadcrumbs.

METHOD.—Cut celery into pieces and cook till tender. Mix cheese with milk. Place celery in a greased baking dish, pour mixture over, cover thickly with breadcrumbs, add a few bits of butter and bake until lightly browned.

BAKED BEETROOT

INGREDIENTS and METHOD.—Wash and prepare in the same way as potatoes that are to be baked in their jackets. They will take a little longer to cook.

BEETROOT IN BUTTER

INGREDIENTS and METHOD.—Choose medium-sized beetroot. Scrub well and cut into ¼ inch slices. Put into saucepan with 2 ounces butter and cook for ¾ to 1 hour, shaking well from time to time. Serve with the juices and butter with a sprinkling of parsley.

PUMPKIN OR MARROW IN BUTTER

INGREDIENTS and METHOD.—Cook as above for beetroot in butter. Leave pumpkin in its shell if it is not a very old one; otherwise peel it.

LEEKS AU GRATIN

INGREDIENTS.—6 leeks, ½ ounce wholemeal flour, 1 ounce butter, ½ pint stock, 1½ ounces grated cheese, a little salt, breadcrumbs.

METHOD.—Trim roots of leeks to within 1 inch of white part. Wash well in salt water and drain. Cook until tender but not soft. Put butter in saucepan and stir in flour, add stock and stir until it boils. Cook for a few minutes and add a little of the cheese. Place leeks in fireproof dish, cover well with sauce, sprinkle over the remainder of cheese mixed with breadcrumbs. Dot small pieces of butter over the top and bake until browned. Serve very hot. This recipe may be used for fritters: Proceed as before, covering leeks with sauce and leaving to cool and set. Dip each piece in egg and breadcrumbs and fry in butter.

ONION RINGS

INGREDIENTS and METHOD.—Peel Spanish onions, cut into thin rings, dip in milk, then wholemeal flour. Drop into smoking hot fat to brown.

BEETROOT IN BUTTER

INGREDIENTS and METHOD.—Carefully wash beetroot, taking care not to bruise skin; cook until tender, about 1 hour if fair size. Cut into cubes, melt butter and reheat in this, adding the juice of a lemon.

STUFFED ONIONS

INGREDIENTS and METHOD.—Choose large onions and cook in a very little water and some fat. Scoop out same of the centre and finely chop it, adding 1 dessertspoon breadcrumbs, ½ teaspoon chopped parsley or mint, and 1 dessertspoon grated cheese or nuts for each onion. Mix these ingredients with a little vegetable stock flavoured with Marmite. Blend well and stuff onions firmly, having the mixture rounding well over the top of the onions. Return to oven and bake till tender. Serve with baked potato and steamed spinach.

SAVOURY MARROW

INGREDIENTS and METHOD.—Some pieces of marrow. Mince a large raw Spanish onion. Put into saucepan 1 ounce fat. Add onion. Cook for a few minutes to brown them. Grate 1 lb. of young turnips and add. Pour over these a small teacup of milk. Add sliced marrow. Cook all together gently about 45 to 50 minutes. Serve hot.

CREAMED SPROUTS

INGREDIENTS.—1 lb. washed Brussels sprouts, 1 pint of fresh milk, 2 ounces grated cheese.

METHOD.—Butter well a large pudding basin, cut sprouts in half and press them into basin. Beat egg and add to milk, then grated cheese. Pour over sprouts, cover basin and steam 1 hour.

Savoury Vegetable and Meat Substitute Dishes

SAVOURY MIXED GRILL

INGREDIENTS and METHOD.—Take equal parts of milled nuts, brown breadcrumbs and mashed potatoes. Add a little Marmite and powdered thyme for flavouring. Mix together to a stiff paste with beaten egg. Shape into cutlets and place in a well buttered tin together with some whole tomatoes, whole partly cooked carrots, onions and parsnips. Put plenty of butter on the vegetables and brown well. Serve with thick brown gravy.

HARICOT DUMPLINGS

INGREDIENTS and METHOD.—Soak overnight and cook ½ lb. haricot beans, ½ lb. diced carrots, ½ lb. sliced onions. Use 2 quarts water to this amount and simmer together till tender. Add Marmite to flavour. Prepare some small dumplings by mixing ½ lb. of flour, 3 ounces butter, 2 ounces cheese or ground nuts, a little thyme or mixed herbs and chopped parsley to a stiff paste with a little milk. Cook in the soup for 20 minutes, adding more liquid if necessary.

NUT ROAST

METHOD.—Put 2 large cups of hazels and almonds through mill, add 1½ cups wholemeal breadcrumbs, 1 teaspoon celery salt, mix and allow to stand 10 minutes. Add 1 to ½ cups hot water, mix again and bake in well greased dish 1 to ½ hours in moderate oven.

HARICOT SAVOURY

INGREDIENTS.—½ lb. soaked haricot beans, 2 ounces cheese, 2 hard boiled eggs, 1 teaspoon, parsley, 1 small finely chopped onion, 1 teacup Marmite gravy.

METHOD.—Cook beans till tender, strain and place a layer in a buttered dish. Sprinkle with minced parsley and onion. Add half the grated cheese and a little seasoning of sage. Cut one of the eggs into thin slices and arrange over the cheese. Add remainder of the beans. Pour Marmite gravy over all. Add remainder of cheese and bake in moderate oven half hour. When cold arrange alternate slices of the other egg with sprigs of parsley.

RISOTTO

INGREDIENTS.—½ lb. brown unpolished rice, 3 ounces cheese, 3 ounces pine kernels (Brazil or walnuts will do), 4 teaspoons chopped onion, 1 pint stock, 2 ounces butter, large teacup tomato puree, a little seasoning if desired.

METHOD.—Fry onion in butter. Put in rice and toss for 4 minutes; add pine kernels, put in stock and cook slowly for about 20 minutes or until rice is tender. Add 2 ounces cheese and let pan remain on side of fire, uncovered, for 10 minutes. Pour heated puree into buttered dish, lay rice over smoothly, pour on remaining puree, and sprinkle over the rest of the cheese. Bake until slightly brown.

SAVOURY RICE

INGREDIENTS and METHOD.—Slice into a saucepan with a small nut of butter, two or three large, absolutely ripe, skinned tomatoes. Add a little—one quite small—chopped or grated onion. Let this simmer for a few minutes until moist, when add one to one and a half tablespoonfuls of washed, natural brown unpolished rice. See that there is sufficient moisture to cook the rice. Simmer together, stirring occasionally, until cooked—about ¾ to one hour—not less. A change is possible by cooking the rice first with a very little sliced onion; and adding, just before serving, one or two tablespoonfuls of minced parsley.

CELERY PIE

INGREDIENTS.—2 heads celery, 1 dessertspoonful butter, mashed potatoes, 1 pint milk, 2 heaped teaspoons of wholemeal flour.

METHOD.—Cook celery till tender—cook and mash potatoes with a little hot milk. Make a sauce of the milk, butter and flour. Put cooked celery into a greased pie-dish, and pour over it the sauce. Cover with mashed potato decorated with chopped parsley or grated onion. Put dabs of butter on top, and bake in oven a nice brown, for about ¾ to 1 hour.

CHEESE CUTLETS

INGREDIENTS.—6 ounces grated cheese, teaspoon mixed mustard, 3 ounces butter, 2 egg yolks.

METHOD.—Mix the cheese, butter, mustard and egg yolks together into a smooth paste. Add salt and cayenne to taste, and stir over the fire until well blended. Put the mixture on a plate to cool, then divide into equal portions, and form into small cutlet shapes.

Whip the whites of the eggs, dip each cutlet in, then coat thickly with breadcrumbs. Insert a small stick of macaroni to take the place of a bone and fry gently in deep fat until nicely browned. Serve very hot.

ALMOND CUTLETS

INGREDIENTS. — ¼ lb. butter beans, 2 ounces almonds, 2 eggs, 1 teaspoon butter.

METHOD. — Rub soaked and cooked beans through sieve and add almonds blanched and put through mill. Add one of the eggs, beaten, and pinch salt; mix thoroughly. Add cited butter and enough wholemeal breadcrumbs to make it possible to mould into cutlets. Shape into about six cutlets, dip each in egg and breadcrumbs and bake in oven.

RICE LOAF

INGREDIENTS. — 2 cups cooked brown rice, 2 cups milled nuts, 4 cups cottage cheese, 4 tablespoons melted butter, 2 teaspoons celery salt.

METHOD. — Mix well, mould into loaf and bake 35-40 minutes.

NUT AND VEGETABLE RISSOLES

INGREDIENTS. — 1 large breakfast cup mixed milled nuts, 1 breakfast cup each grated raw carrot, turnip, celeriac, 1½ breakfast cups, cold, well mashed potato, 2 finely chopped onions, ½ teaspoon dried mixed herbs, ½ teaspoon celery salt.

METHOD. — Mix well and bind with an egg. Form into rissoles, roll in breadcrumbs or oatmeal and bake in medium oven until brown.

NUT CUTLETS

INGREDIENTS. — 4 breakfast cups wholemeal breadcrumbs, 3 cups milled nuts, ½ cup minced onion, ½ cup parsley, 2 eggs.

METHOD. — Shape and bake 1 hour. Serve with tomato sauce.

NUT CROQUETTES

INGREDIENTS and METHOD.—Mix well 1 cup milled nuts (walnuts, almonds, filberts or Brazils), 1 cup wholemeal breadcrumbs soaked in ½ cup of milk, 1 egg, seasoning to taste. Shape and brown in oven.

STUFFED NUT ROAST

INGREDIENTS.—4 steamed onions, 6 ounces wholemeal breadcrumbs, 2 ounces fat, ½ teaspoon Marmite, 1 dessertspoon hot stock, 1 dessertspoon powdered sage, ½ cup milled nuts, 1 well beaten egg. 2 ounces onion cream, 3 ounces Soyolk (soya flour).

METHOD.—Chop onions very fine and beat in other ingredients, dust board with milled nuts, stir together the dry ingredients, make a hole and pour in beaten egg and stock. Mix to a stiff paste. Roll out and fill with the stuffing, like a sandwich. Brush each side before stuffing and before adding top layer, with egg, brush outside also to prevent loss of moisture. Bake well 20-30 minutes.

Stuffing: Chop onions well and beat in other seasonings; work to right consistency with small amount of stock.

RICE CHEESE SAVOURY

INGREDIENTS.—4 ounces rice, 4 ounces cheese, butter, 2 beaten eggs, ½ pint milk, nutmeg.

METHOD.—Soak rice overnight in boiling water; then wash well. Cook, butter it, then mix in ⅔ cheese, half quantity of egg and any herbs or seasoning that is liked. Pour rest of egg, cheese and milk over top and dust with nutmeg. Bake till lightly browned.

SUMMER STEW

INGREDIENTS. — 1 bunch of young carrots, 3 or 4 young turnips, 1 large minced onion, 2 tablespoons of seedless raisins or sultanas, water or vegetable stock, 1 lb. shelled peas,.1 large sweet ripe apple, 1 large tablespoon of brown gage, 1½ ounces nut fat, chopped mint.

METHOD. — Melt fat in a casserole dish, add stock and cook minced onions 10 minutes. Now add carrots cut in long thin strips, the turnips (grated), then raisins and sago. Just cover with stock. When it comes to the boil add peas and chopped apple. Cook gently half to one hour.

CAULIFLOWER, TOMATO AND CHEESE CASSEROLE

INGREDIENTS. — 1 large cauliflower, 1 cup grated cheese; 4 large tomatoes, butter, wholemeal breadcrumbs, minced onion, ¾ pint milk, flour.

METHOD. — Steam cauliflower and break into sprigs, slice tomatoes. Make a sauce of flour, butter, milk and seasoning and add onions, which have been cooked in a little butter. Put alternate layers of cauliflower, tomato, cheese, breadcrumbs and sauce into a casserole dish, finishing with breadcrumbs, and bake in moderate oven 35 to 40 minutes.

NUT AND VEGETABLE ROAST

INGREDIENTS. — 1 cup grated carrot, 1 cup bread crumbs, 1 egg, ½ cup milled nuts, 1 tablespoon butter, 1 cup strained tomato, onion to taste.

METHOD. — Mix, shape into loaf and steam 1 hour, then brown in oven.

COMPOTE VEGETABLES AND FORCEMEAT

INGREDIENTS.—1 lb. new potatoes, 1 lb. young peas (shelled), 1½ lb. new turnips and carrots (mixed), 2 Spanish onions or large bunch spring onions, 2 tablespoons wholemeal flour, mint.

METHOD.—Dice turnips and carrots, shell peas, leave potatoes whole. Place all in saucepan, just cover with vegetable stock and bring to boil. Throw in mint. Turn gas very low and simmer for ¼ hour.

Prepare forcemeat balls as follows:

INGREDIENTS.—3 ounces nuts (walnuts), 3 ounces brown breadcrumbs, 1 dessertspoon of oil, 1 egg.

METHOD.—Mix nuts, herbs, breadcrumbs and onions together, stir in oil and bind with beaten egg. Roll into little balls with plenty of wholemeal flour. When vegetables have cooked, stir in one teaspoon of Marmite. Drop in forcemeat balls and cook gently another 25 to 30 minutes.. When done take out forcemeat balls and potatoes and arrange round dish and keep hot. Sprinkle flour into saucepan, stir a few minutes. When compote is thick, dish in centre of potatoes, etc. Forcemeat balls can be cooked separately in deep fat and served with any conservatively cooked vegetables.

VEGETABLE ROAST

INGREDIENTS.—¼ cup melted butter, 1½ cups milled nuts, 3 eggs, 2 tablespoons minced onions, ½ cup of milk, or enough to moisten sufficiently, 1 cup celery cut fine, 3 cups wholemeal breadcrumbs, 1 tablespoon minced parsley, little salt and Marmite.

METHOD.—Mix all well together, form into loaf, bake in moderate oven about an hour. Baste with melted butter and water mixed.

SUMMER VEGETABLES MEDLEY

INGREDIENTS. — 1 cauliflower (small), 1 bunch young carrots, 3 or 4 young turnips, 1 lb. new peas (shelled), 3 or 4 new potatoes, 1 tablespoon of pot barley, finely chopped mint to taste.

METHOD. — Divide cauliflower into small pieces, leave carrots whole if small, if not cut lengthwise, turnips cut in circles, potatoes in cubes, shelled peas, chopped mint. Place all vegetables in a casserole dish, cauliflower at the bottom, then carrots, turnips, peas, potatoes, with the barley on top and lastly the mint. Pour in sufficient boiling water to barely cover the vegetables, put on lid, and cook very gently until all moisture is absorbed. Look from time to time to make sure water has not cooked away too soon. Add more as required. Serve with coddled eggs, cream cheese or any of the simple egg or cheese dishes. Dry toasted bread, or or baked bread, or Rye-Vita biscuits make the hard food.

NUT MEAT SUPREME

INGREDIENTS. — 6 ounces of milled mixed nuts, 2 ounces toasted brown breadcrumbs, 1 teaspoon of mixed herbs, ½ ounce nut fat, ½ gill (70m ml) of vegetable stock, 2 ounces cooked mashed potatoes, 2 ounces cooked brown rice, ½ teaspoon of powdered sage, 1 minced raw onion, 1 egg.

METHOD. — Mix herbs and celery salt into nuts, add breadcrumbs and onions, work potato in smoothly, warm fat and mix in. Beat egg and mix in the stock and mix all to a firm paste. Be careful not to make it too wet. Put into greased basin and steam 30 minutes. Leave in basin to cool. Turn out. Use next day if possible as it cuts better.

CAULIFLOWER AND NUT PIE

INGREDIENTS.—1 large cauliflower, ½ teacup grated cheese, ½ teacup minced nuts, ½ pint thick sauce made with wholemeal flour, butter and milk.

METHOD.—For potato crust: ½ lb. potatoes cooked in their jackets and mashed after peeling, 4 ounces wholemeal flour, 2 ounces butter, little milk. Wash the cauliflower and boil it gently until tender, then break into neat flowerettes and place in a greased casserole dish or pie-dish. Cover with the nuts and grated cheese, and pour over all the lettuce.

Mix the flour with the mashed potato; rub in butter; add seasoning to taste and enough cold milk to make easily handled and formed into a paste. Roll out on floured board about ½-inch thick; cover the cauliflower, etc., and bake in moderate oven about half an hour.

POTATOES WITH CHEESE

INGREDIENTS and METHOD.—Boil in their jackets one pound of potatoes. Mash them and add 2 tablespoonfuls of butter, a little wholemeal breadcrumbs soaked in milk, and three tablespoonfuls of grated cheese. Beat to a smooth, fairly stiff consistency. Add the lightly whisked yolks of 2 eggs, a dessertspoon of chopped parsley and a little pepper and salt. Lastly add the egg whites stiffly whisked. Put into a greased pie-dish, smooth the top and brush over with melted butter. Do not fill dish too full as the mixture rises. Bake in a moderate oven for an hour and a quarter. It should be light, nicely set and golden.

CAULIFLOWER ROAST

INGREDIENTS. — 1 large cauliflower, ½ lb. of milled Brazil nuts, 1 meagre cupful of wholemeal breadcrumbs, 1 ounce butter, 3 or 4 tablespoons of strong onion stock.

METHOD. — Partly cook cauliflower, break into small pieces and pile on to a greased dish (baking dish). Melt fat, mix with breadcrumbs, stock and nuts to make a stiff paste. Cover the cauliflower with this mixture and cover again with a layer of toasted crumbs or Corn flakes. Dot with butter. Bake quickly to brown.

POTATOES AU GRATIN

INGREDIENTS. — 2 lb. potatoes, 1 tablespoon breadcrumbs, 1½ teaspoons wholemeal flour, 4 tablespoons grated cheese, 1 tablespoon finely minced onion, a little butter.

METHOD. — Wash and boil potatoes in their jackets. Peel and cut into slices. Butter a pie-dish, put in a layer of potatoes, sprinkle with a little onion and cheese, then another layer of potatoes and so on. Mix the flour with 1 gill (140 ml) of milk or vegetable stock and pour over all. Sprinkle top with breadcrumbs and dot with butter. Bake half an hour.

ONION TART

INGREDIENTS and METHOD. — Line a shallow dish with short crust. Cut up a bunch or two of spring onions, or ordinary onions, brown in butter and add a pinch of salt. Remove from fire and stir in 3 eggs and 3 large tablespoons thick cream, and when well mixed pour into the pastry. Cook in hot oven for half an hour.

BROAD BEAN PIE

INGREDIENTS. — 2lb. young beans, 1 large Spanish onion, shredded, a little fresh sage or half a teaspoon of dried sage.

METHOD. — Cook all together, allowing just enough water to make a little gravy when done. When nearly cooked turn into pie-dish and add ¼ teaspoon of Marmite to the juice. Make following mixture and place on top of beans, adding a finishing layer of Corn flakes or breadcrumbs, and bake for half an hour.

Mixture: 3 tablespoons of wholemeal flour, yolks of 2 eggs, 2 tablespoons of grated cheese. Mix flour with milk and egg yolks well beaten, and lastly cheese. Make this of a creamy consistency.

CELERY LOAF

INGREDIENTS. — 1 small cup wholemeal breadcrumbs, cup minced parsley, 1 large minced onion, 2 eggs, well beaten, pinch of whole spice, 1½ cups diced celery, ¾ cup walnuts, ground finely, 4 small mushrooms (if in season), 1 teaspoon butter, 1½ cups milk.

METHOD. — Mix well, stand 20 minutes. Bake in moderate oven for half an hour.

MUSHROOM CUTLETS

INGREDIENTS. — 2 lb. mushrooms, 2 ounces wholemeal flour, 2 eggs, 4 ounces wholemeal breadcrumbs.

METHOD. — Peel and chop mushrooms and mix the flour and breadcrumbs well together. Add the mushrooms to these with a little salt. Add beaten eggs and a little milk if necessary. Form into cutlets and dip in egg and baked breadcrumbs, and fry in olive oil until golden brown. Serve very hot with slices of lemon.

MACARONI AND NUT CUTLETS

INGREDIENTS. — ¼ lb. wholemeal macaroni, ¼ lb. milled walnuts, 1 egg, 1 onion, 1 dessertspoon finely chopped parsley, ½ cup Marmite stock.

METHOD. — Put macaroni into boiling water and cook. Then mince it. Add nuts, the minced and browned onion, beaten egg, parsley, etc. Mix all together well. Form into cutlets, brush with a little of the beaten egg and breadcrumbs (dextrinised) and bake in oven, or fry in butter.

MACARONI CHEESE

INGREDIENTS and METHOD. — Boil 3 ounces macaroni in quickly boiling water, slightly salted. Drain well. Make sauce of ½ pint of milk, 1 gill (140 ml) of water in which the wholemeal macaroni was cooked, 1 ounce wholemeal flour, and 2 ounces butter. Add the macaroni, a teaspoon of made mustard, a little finely minced onion, 4 ounces grated cheese and seasonings. When well mixed pour into a well greased fireproof dish, sprinkle with a little cheese (about an ounce), some breadcrumbs, and pour over a little melted butter. Brown in oven.

NUT MEAT

INGREDIENTS. — ½ cup each of walnuts, Brazils, and almonds minced, ½ cup peanut butter, 2 cups wholemeal flour, 1 onion, enough boiling water to moisten the whole.

METHOD. — Let stand for 10 minutes and then add 1 cup of cold water with 1 egg beaten into it and mix. well. Flavour with a little celery salt, put into an oiled dish and bake for 1 hour in moderate oven. Serve either hot or cold. If hot, serve with brown gravy.

CHEESE AND POTATO ROAST

INGREDIENTS.—1 cupful grated cheese, ½ lb. potatoes cooked in jackets, then finely mashed, 2 cupfuls wholemeal breadcrumbs, 1 egg, onion flavouring.

METHOD.—Mix well together, bind with egg, press firmly together, sprinkle with flour and bake for half an hour.

DUTCH PIE

INGREDIENTS.—6 potatoes, 1 onion, 4 ounces of cheese, teacup of breadcrumbs, 1 breakfast cup of milk, 1 dessertspoon of butter, seasoning.

METHOD.—Grease dish, dust over with breadcrumbs and cheese. Mix rest of crumbs and cheese, onion and salt. Slice potatoes finely and fill dish with alternate layers. Dot over with butter, pour milk over, steam or bake 1 hour.

GRANOSE CHEESE SAVOURY

INGREDIENTS.—2 breakfast cups of Corn flakes, 2 eggs, 4 ounces grated cheese, ¾ pint of milk.

METHOD.—Mix flakes and cheese together, beat eggs and add milk, stir in flakes, place in buttered dish and bake till brown.

GRANOSE GLOBES

INGREDIENTS.—1 breakfast cup of strained mashed potatoes, 1 teacup of Corn flakes, 1 teacup of dry Cheddar cheese, 1 egg.

METHOD.—Mix all together, add beaten egg, and if necessary a little milk. Form into balls in plenty of oatmeal, fry in deep fat or bake in hot oven till slightly brown.

STEAMED NUT SAVOURY

INGREDIENTS. — 1 shredded wheat biscuit, 2 ounces milled Brazils, 2 ounces milled walnuts or peanuts, 1 small egg to bind mixture, 5 tablespoons of strong vegetable stock, flavoured with ¼ teaspoon of Marmite if liked.

METHOD. — Break up shredded wheat into fine crumbs and cover with the heated stock. When the crumbs are softened stir in the nuts. Bind with whisked egg. Place in buttered dish and steam 30 minutes. Can be eaten hot or cold.

TOKYO SAVOURY

INGREDIENTS. — ½ cup of brown rice, 1 large onion, 1 breakfast cup grated Cheddar cheese, 1 egg, 1 shredded Wheat Biscuit or toast crumbs, water.

METHOD. — Wash rice very well, place in double boiler, cover with boiling water, add raw onion chopped very small, and cook till grains separate and onion is quite tender. Turn into bowl, add cheese, and mix with well beaten egg. Sprinkle crumbs over mixture. Bake in hot oven 20 minutes.

SICILIAN SAVOURY

INGREDIENTS. — 1 dessertspoon of nut oil, 3 large Spanish onions, 4 ounces of egg vermicelli, 4 ounces grated cheese, 1 tablespoon of brown breadcrumbs, 3 medium-sized tomatoes, 3 tablespoons of vegetable stock.

METHOD. — Mince onions, skin tomatoes, break up vermicelli. Pour oil and stock into saucepan, add onions, etc., and cook gently until soft. Add breadcrumbs and cheese. Stir a few minutes merely to heat through. Serve on very hot dish, sprinkle with parsley and rest of cheese.

NUT MEAT SUPREME

INGREDIENTS. — 6 ounces of milled mixed nuts, 2 ounces toasted brown breadcrumbs, 1 teaspoon of mixed herbs, ½ ounce nut fat, ½ gill (70m ml) of vegetable stock, 2 ounces cooked mashed potatoes, 2 ounces cooked brown rice, ½ teaspoon of powdered sage, 1 minced raw onion, 1 egg.

METHOD. — Mix herbs and celery salt into nuts, add breadcrumbs and onions, work potato in smoothly, warm fat and mix in. Beat egg and mix in the stock and mix all to a firm paste. Be careful not to make it too wet. Put into greased basin and steam 30 minutes. Leave in basin to cool. Turn out. Use next day if possible as it cuts better.

SAVOURY RABBIT*

INGREDIENTS and METHOD. — Soak rabbits in salted water 1 hour. Dry well, cut into neat joints and coat with wholemeal flour and seasoning. Place in casserole dish with sliced onions. Cover with milk; put on lid and gently bake in oven 1½ hours. Prepare a forcemeat, remove lid from casserole dish and pour off a little of the milk, cover rabbit with forcemeat and bake in oven 1 hour more without lid.

Forcemeat: 4 ounces wholemeal breadcrumbs, 2 ounces butter, 1 teaspoon parsley, ½ teaspoon mixed dried herbs, a little salt and 1 beaten egg. This may be varied by substituting 1 teaspoon grated lemon rind, or 1 teaspoon chopped onion, 3 or 4 sage leaves or tomato sauce.

VEGETABLE SAVOURY

INGREDIENTS.—2 large parsnips, 2 ounces cottage cheese (home made), chopped parsley, wholemeal breadcrumbs, ½ pint vegetable stock, a little grated Cheddar cheese.

METHOD.—Cook and mash parsnips, add cottage cheese, sprinkle wholemeal flour or crumbs on board, lay mixture on and shape into cakes about an inch thick. Roll thickly in grated cheese and grill on both sides. Serve with vegetable stock boiled up with diced carrot or beetroot flavoured with minced onion; or with brown sauce.

HOME-MADE CHEESE

To 1 pint milk, preferably from the day before, add 2 teaspoons lemon juice. Stir with wooden spoon. Heat very gently in enamel saucepan. Strain through muslin. Break up curd and if possible add a little cream. A little finely grated onion, or tomato pulp, finely grated cheese, parsley or mint make a variety of flavours. This is specially suitable to serve with vegetables and salads.

NUT SURPRISE

INGREDIENTS.—2 cups of breadcrumbs, ¼ cupful of walnuts, ¼ cupful of Barcelonas, cupful of peanuts, ¼ cups of boiled rice, ¼ cupful of almonds, 6 hard-boiled eggs, 3 raw eggs, 1 teaspoon of grated onion, seasoning.

METHOD.—Put breadcrumbs into saucepan, cover with water and boil 5 minutes. Remove from fire and add nuts which have been milled or minced. Then add rice, hard boiled eggs chopped fine, seasoning, etc. Stir well, add raw eggs well beaten. Shape into loaf. Brush with butter and bake in moderate oven 1 hour. Serve very hot.

VEGETABLE CURRY

INGREDIENTS and METHOD.—Fry 1 large apple and onion finely sliced. Cook till tender and add about 1½ cups milk or stock, a little salt and seasoning, 1 teaspoon sugar and small piece butter and 1 dessertspoon curry powder. Stir well and bring to the boil. Now add any left over vegetables—cooked peas, beans, parsnips, celery, cabbage, etc.—or one kind alone makes a very savoury dish. Mix in a little wholemeal flour. Heat vegetables through thoroughly and serve very hot. If liked a border of boiled brown rice may be served round the curry.

BEAN, CARROT AND PEANUT LOAF

INGREDIENTS.—1 cup each grated raw carrot and thick bean pulp, ¼ cup peanut butter, 1 cup wholemeal breadcrumbs, 1 cup tomatoes, 1 cup boiled brown rice, 2 tablespoons butter, ¼ teaspoon mustard, ½ small onion, minced; a little minced celery, seasoning according to taste.

METHOD.—Mix in given order and shape into loaf. Bake about 45 minutes.

CABBAGE AND CHEESE PIE

INGREDIENTS.—1 lb. shredded cabbage, 4 tablespoons butter, 4 tablespoons wholemeal flour, 2 cups milk, 1 teaspoon salt, ½ lb. Cheddar cheese, 1½ cups broken spaghetti.

METHOD.—Cook spaghetti in boiling salted water till tender. Drain well. Melt butter in saucepan, stir in flour and when frothy stir in milk. Keep stirring till smooth; then season and add cheese. Place cabbage, spaghetti and sauce in layers in a buttered dish; cover with wholemeal breadcrumbs and dot with butter. Bake from ¾ hour in moderate oven.

NUT AND VEGETABLE PIE

INGREDIENTS and METHOD.—One cup dried beans which have been soaked and partly cooked (lima, haricot, or navy beans will do), 2 turnips, 1 head of celery, 6 mushrooms, if obtainable, 2 carrots, 1 large onion, 1 cup milk, mashed potato and ½ lb. finely chopped nuts. Put partly cooked beans, carrots, turnips, celery and onion into milk and stew gently until tender. Prepare mushrooms and place them on top of vegetables in a pie-dish. Sprinkle over a little chopped parsley and add a small piece of butter. Cover with a thick covering of mashed potatoes dotted with butter. Cover with chopped or milled nuts and bake till brown. Serve very hot with melted butter sauce.

COTTAGE CHEESE

INGREDIENTS and METHOD.—Set 1 quart of milk, and skim off the cream. Save cream. Make an ordinary junket without sweetening, with the skimmed milk. When junket has set break up with a fork and heat slowly over a low gas. Stir with fork until the whey separates from the curd—this takes only a few minutes; remove from gas, and drain off the whey. Leave to stand for a few hours, then mash curd up with a fork, and add some of the cream which was saved. This curd gives a generous helping for four people.

Savoury Moulds and Jellies

GELAZONE GALANTINE

INGREDIENTS.—6 ounces milled walnuts, 3 ounces wholemeal breadcrumbs, 1 egg, 1 gill (140 ml) milk, medium minced onion.

METHOD.—Mix and steam 1 hour in greased basin. Cut into cubes when cold. For Jelly: Pint strong vegetable stock, gelo or gelatine or agar agar, 1 teaspoon sage tied in muslin, Marmite. Pour this over alternate layers of cubed peas, carrots or any other suitable cooked vegetable. Decorate with parsley and serve with green salad.

SAVOURY TOMATO JELLY

INGREDIENTS.—1 lb. fresh tomatoes, 1 teaspoon agar agar, small minced onion, 2 ounces sago, ½ pint strong vegetable stock, ½ gill (70 ml) cold water, 6 ounces ground walnuts, 1 ounce butter.

METHOD.—Cook skinned tomatoes, sago, butter and stock. Then beat well with fork over pot of boiling water with the agar. Remove, add onion and nuts, set, decorate, and serve with salad.

CHEESE MOULD

INGREDIENTS.—4 medium-sized tomatoes, 1½ ounces breadcrumbs, 3 ounces cheese, 1 tablespoon agar agar, ½ pint strong vegetable stock, minced onion or leek.

METHOD.—Mash skinned tomatoes and gradually add cheese, then breadcrumbs. Dissolve the agar or gelatine in the stock, add all ingredients. Set and serve with salad.

LENTIL AND RICE MOULD

INGREDIENTS.—1½ cups lentils, 1 cup rice, 1 grated onion, 1 teaspoon mixed herbs, 2 tablespoons butter, 1 teaspoon salt.

METHOD.—Cook rice and lentils together, add other ingredients, steam in buttered basin 1½ hours, turn out when cold, garnish and serve with salad.

SAVOURY JELLY

INGREDIENTS and METHOD.—Make a strong soup by simmering onions, carrots, parsnips, etc. Add a little parsley or sage, dissolve sufficient gelatine and add to strained stock. Serve cold.

SAVOURY BRAWN

INGREDIENTS.—1 pint strong vegetable stock, 2 ounces steamed carrots cut into tiny dice, 2 ounces wholemeal macaroni, good teaspoon Marmite, Nut Meat Supreme as given in this book, sufficient gelatine to set.

METHOD.—Prepare macaroni by breaking up into small pieces and cooking in barely 1 gill (140 ml) water 10 to 15 minutes. Pour stock into double boiler, add Marmite and gelatine and cook gently till dissolved. Wet a mould and put in alternate layers of carrots, macaroni and nut meat; continue till basin is three parts filled. Pour jelly liquid over all, cover closely and set aside to cool. Green peas and broad beans may be used with advantage instead of macaroni.

Egg Dishes, Soufflés, Omelettes, Savoury Batters, and Pancakes

CHEESE TART

INGREDIENTS.—1 ounce butter, 2 eggs, ¾ ounce wholemeal flour, ¼ pint milk, 2 ounces grated cheese. Salt, pepper and a little mustard or cayenne.

METHOD.—Melt the butter in a pan, mix well with the flour, then add the milk and boil. Add the grated cheese, egg yolks, and seasonings. Lastly stir in the egg whites beaten stiffly, one at a time. Line a shallow tin with short crust made with wholemeal flour and butter, pour in mixture and bake till set and brown.

SPINACH SOUFFLÉ

INGREDIENTS.—1 lb. cooked spinach, 3 eggs, ½ ounce butter, 2 tablespoons cream.

METHOD.—Steam spinach and rub through sieve, add yolks and cream, then stiffly beaten whites. Sprinkle with a few wholemeal breadcrumbs and bake ¼ hour.

CARROT SHAPE WITH GREAT PEAS

INGREDIENTS and METHOD.—2 cups cooked and finely mashed carrot, add a little seasoning to taste and some finely shredded onion and three eggs beaten with a cup of rich milk. Put into a well buttered pyrex dish, and push a small basin down the middle, and bake gently until the egg mixture is set. Lift out the basin and fill hollow with freshly cooked green peas, sprinkled with finely chopped mint.

CHEESE AND TOMATO SOUFFLÉ

INGREDIENTS. — ¼ lb. butter, 4 eggs, ¼ lb. wholemeal flour, ¼ lb. cheese, ½ pint milk, 4 tomatoes.

METHOD. — Skin and chop tomatoes. Make sauce of butter, flour and milk. Mix in yolks and cheese, add beaten whites, pour over tomatoes and bake in hot oven 15 to 20 minutes.

ONION SOUFFLÉ

INGREDIENTS. — 2 tablespoons of flour (wholemeal), 3 tablespoons butter, 3 tablespoons cheese (finely grated), 3 eggs, ¾ pint of milk, 2 pounds onions.

METHOD. — Peel and chop onions fairly fine and stew for 10 minutes in the butter, add a little salt. Make the cheese, milk and flour into a sauce, using some of the milk to mix the flour with. Cook for a few minutes. Take off the fire and stir in the egg yolks and when quite cold and just before putting into the oven, the stiffly beaten white. Put the onions into a deep dish or casserole dish and pour over the sauce. Bake 25 to 35 minutes.

GREEN PEA SOUFFLÉ

Same as Onion Soufflé.

FRENCH BEAN SOUFFLÉ

Same as Onion Soufflé.

CAULIFLOWER SOUFFLÉ

Same as Onion Soufflé.

SWISS EGGS

INGREDIENTS and METHOD.—Line a shallow dish with grated cheese, and pour in a mixture of 1 cup of milk, 1 beaten egg, salt, pepper, mustard to taste. Break in as many eggs as required and bake for 10 minutes or so in hot oven.

VEGETABLE SOUFFLÉ

INGREDIENTS.—1 or 2 cauliflowers, 2 lb. potatoes, 2½ ounces butter, 2½ ounces flour, 2 pints vegetable stock and milk, 4 ounces cheese, little cream, 3 eggs.

METHOD.—Steam cauliflower till only just soft. Cook potatoes in jackets and peel. Slice thinly and put in dish. Sprinkle with half the cheese. Break cauliflower, and put on potatoes, cover with sauce of butter, flour, milk stock, cream and beaten eggs. Sprinkle with cheese and butter. Cook in hot oven ½ to ¾ hour till brown crust is formed.

SPINACH ENTREE

INGREDIENTS.—1 lb. spinach, 4 ounces wholemeal breadcrumbs, 2 tomatoes, 1 large onion, 4 ounces grated cheese, ½ pint stock and milk, 2 eggs.

METHOD.—Steam spinach and chop finely, skin and chop tomatoes, mince onions. Mix these with the breadcrumbs, stock and cheese. Add yolks and mix well. Whisk whites very stiff and fold in. Bake in greased dish till firmly set.

EGGS AND GRANOSE

INGREDIENTS and METHOD.—Two tablespoons Corn flakes and a little butter. Break egg on to this; set in oven; serve with greens and carrots.

SPINACH OMELETTE

INGREDIENTS. — 2 tablespoons cooked spinach for each person, 1 ounce butter, 2 eggs.

METHOD. — Before folding omelette over place spinach as hot and dry as possible on top, fold and finish cooking about another minute.

WALNUT OMELETTE

INGREDIENTS. — 2 eggs, 2 tablespoons milk, 2 dessertspoons chopped walnuts, 1 dessertspoon seedless raisins.

METHOD. — Beat eggs very thoroughly, add milk and beat again. Melt some butter in pan. Mix nuts into eggs and milk lightly and quickly. Pour in pan and stir till cooked. Toss out, sprinkle with raisins, fold over and serve with spinach or other green vegetable.

VEGETABLE OMELETTE

INGREDIENTS. — 2 eggs, butter, 2 or 3 tomatoes, sliced and grilled, green peas (about a cupful), 2 carrots, cooked and diced.

METHOD. — Beat white and yolks separately and mix together. Heat butter and pour in eggs; cook till set. Place some of the peas, carrots and tomato on top, fold over, and serve with rest of vegetables.

SYLVAN EGGS

INGREDIENTS and METHOD. — Line a greased pie-dish with hot mashed potatoes, add a layer of hot mashed carrot, then one of hot minced onion. Break in 1 egg for each person, sprinkle with butter and chopped parsley and breadcrumbs, cover with another pie-dish and bake till eggs are set.

BREADCRUMB AND ONION OMELETTE WITH CHEESE SAUCE

INGREDIENTS.—4 eggs, 1 cup wholemeal breadcrumbs, 1 onion, ½ pint milk, 1 ounce cheese, ½ ounce butter.

METHOD.—Sauce: Melt the butter and stir in flour, 1 tablespoonful. Add slowly ½ pint milk. Stir till smooth and cooked; then add cheese. Soak the breadcrumbs in equal quantities of milk and water and then drain them. Brown finely chopped onion in butter. Mix breadcrumbs and yolks and lightly fold in well beaten whites. Pour the mixture over onions, cover and cook gently. Serve folded over with sauce poured round. If mushrooms are procurable they may be chopped, fried and added to the sauce.

FRICASSEE OF EGGS

INGREDIENTS.—4 eggs, 4 tomatoes, 1 pint white sauce, 2 tablespoons wholemeal breadcrumbs, 1 teaspoon chopped parsley, 1 ounce butter, seasoning.

METHOD.—Hard boil eggs and cut into quarters; add to sauce and heat through gently. Cut tomatoes in halves, sprinkle with salt and crumbs, put a little butter on each and bake till tender. Put eggs on dish, sprinkle parsley over, arrange tomatoes round and serve very hot.

BOMBAY EGGS

INGREDIENTS.—1 egg, a pinch of curry powder, 3 tablespoons cooked rice, spinach.

METHOD.—Break egg into basin and stand in bowl of hot water half-way up. When egg begins to set stir in curry powder quickly, but gently. Put the hot rice surrounded with spinach on to plate, turn egg on top. Have egg just creamy.

CURRIED EGG RISSOLES

INGREDIENTS.—4 hard boiled eggs, 4 ounces breadcrumbs, 2 ounces Soyolk (soya flour), 1 grated raw apple, 1 beaten egg, ¾ teaspoon Marmite, 1 dessertspoon curry powder, hot vegetable stock to mix.

METHOD.—Grate in to the breadcrumbs the eggs; add all other ingredients and bind with egg. Shape into rissoles, brush with egg, fry in deep fat.

EGG CUTLETS

INGREDIENTS.—3 eggs, ½ pint of milk, 1 ounce butter, 2 ounces flour, breadcrumbs.

METHOD.—Boil eggs well until just hard, and put through sieve. Make a sauce with other ingredients, sufficiently thick to stand in balls when mixed with eggs. Allow to get cold. Shape into cutlets, dip in egg and breadcrumbs, Cook in very hot fat 2 minutes.

TOMATO EGGS

INGREDIENTS and METHOD.—1 large tomato, cut in half and cooked gently in a casserole dish. Take from casserole dish and scoop out pulp, drop raw egg inside. Return to casserole dish and cook till egg is set. Make sauce of pulp with stock, flour, etc. Serve with spinach and carrots.

BAKED EGGS

INGREDIENTS and METHOD.—Butter individual dishes, add 1 tablespoon milk to each, sprinkle with chopped chives, parsley or onion; break in egg; sprinkle with wholemeal breadcrumbs and bake.

EGG AND POTATO PIE

INGREDIENTS.—1 lb. potatoes, 2 ounces grated cheese, 6 hard boiled eggs, ½ pint wholemeal flour sauce.

METHOD.—Leave boiled potatoes till quite cold. Fill a dish with alternate layers sliced potatoes and sliced egg. Sprinkle cheese between layers and season. Pour over sauce, sprinkle with thin layer of cheese and brown in oven.

EGG AND LENTIL SAVOURY

INGREDIENTS.—4 ounces lentils, 2 roast onions, 1 grated hard boiled egg, 1 tomato, butter, casserole vegetables.

METHOD.—Cook lentils quickly in stock. When vegetables and lentils are ready place vegetables in pie-dish. Make a crust of egg and lentils. Chop tomato and onion finely, add a little butter and a little Marmite dissolved in hot water, mix with tomato and onion and add these to vegetables, in dish. Cover with lentil crust, brush with egg and bake.

SAVOURY BATTER (3 to 4 people)

INGREDIENTS.—¼ lb. wholemeal flour, 1 pint of milk, 3 new laid eggs, 2 raw and minced Spanish onions, ½ teaspoon of Marmite.

METHOD.—Pour flour into bowl, make well in middle and break the eggs into the hollow. Beat with fork thoroughly. Melt Marmite in just a little of the milk, then add to cold milk, gradually working it into the batter until all is smooth. Mix in minced onion. If mixture can stand for an hour or even 30 minutes the result will be better. Pour mixture into well greased dish and bake in moderate oven 10 to 50 minutes.

SAVOURY EGGS

INGREDIENTS and METHOD. — Eggs poached in small moulds with parsley and cheese sprinkled at bottom. Serve with spinach or chopped buttered cabbage, or turnip, but if turnips are used serve also some green or juicy vegetable or marrow, runner beans, onions, cabbage, etc.

Fish Dishes

SAVOURY FISH FLAN

INGREDIENTS and METHOD.—Butter a pie-dish and put in fillets of fish; season and sprinkle with lemon juice. Melt 1 ounce butter, mix in 2 tablespoons wholemeal flour, 1 teaspoon chopped parsley, 1 teaspoon curry powder. Work in 2 beaten eggs and ½ pint milk. Pour over fish. Stand pie-dish in a tin of water and bake in moderate oven for half hour.

FISH WITH LEMON SAUCE

INGREDIENTS and METHOD.—2 lb. white fish. Put 1½ breakfast cups milk and small onion in a pan and when almost boiling add fish cut in pieces. Simmer till fish is lender, about 10 minutes. Remove fish and onion, add beaten egg with juice and rind of half a lemon. Stir till it thickens. Pour over fish and decorate with parsley. May be eaten hot or cold.

FISH SALAD

INGREDIENTS and METHOD.—2 lb. cold steamed fish in small pieces. Line salad bowl with lettuce leaves, pile fish In centre. Cover with mayonnaise and decorate with parsley. Round base of fish arrange water cress, diced cooked beetroot, sliced tomato and cucumber.

FILLETED FISH WITH MUSHROOMS

INGREDIENTS and METHOD.—Cook mushrooms in butter till tender. Rub fillets with lemon juice. Cool and chop mushrooms; spread on fillets, roll up, cook 20 minutes in a well buttered casserole dish.

FISH SOUFFLÉ

INGREDIENTS.—2 ounces cooked fish, 1 gill (140 ml) milk, 1 teaspoon flour, 1 teaspoon parsley, 1 egg.

METHOD.—Flake fish finely, make sauce of butter, flour and milk. Cook and remove from fire, add seasonings and yolk; add fish, lastly fold in well beaten white. Bake till brown and serve at once. Quantity for one person.

GROPER RAREBIT

INGREDIENTS and METHOD.—Cut 1 lb. groper into fillets; sprinkle with lemon juice. Bake with dots of butter 15 minutes in moderate oven. When nearly done sprinkle over 3 ounces grated cheese and some chopped parsley. Put another once butter into dish and cook till slightly browned.

FISH CURRY

INGREDIENTS.—1 lb. white fish, such as blue cod or groper, 2 ounces butter, 1 small onion, 12 sultanas, 1 tomato, ½ pint milk, 1 large dessertspoon wholemeal flour, salt to taste, teacupful brown rice, 1 teaspoon curry powder.

METHOD.—Wash fish and strip from bone, put into a saucepan with the milk, grated onion, tomato, and a sprinkling of salt. Simmer gently for 20 minutes, then remove from pan, flake. Heat butter and mix flour in smoothly, strain into this the milk in which fish was cooked and stir over gentle heat till it thickens. Mix the curry powder with the fish and stir into sauce; add sultanas.

Boil rice in salted water 20 minutes, drain well and shake, the grains separate; make into a ring on hot dish and pour curry mixture into centre. Garnish lemon and parsley.

SAVOURY FISH

INGREDIENTS and METHOD. — Sprinkle any kind of white fish with a little salt and pepper and place in earthenware dish. Pour over ½ pint milk and ½ pint water. Cover dish, cook slowly in oven till fish is tender. Lift out fish and keep hot. Add 2 tablespoons wholemeal breadcrumbs and 1 ounce of butter to liquid and cook till crumbs swell and sauce thickens. Then add chopped parsley and 3 teaspoons lemon juice, return fish to sauce and serve at once.

BAKED FISH

INGREDIENTS. — 1 fish such as cod or trevally, 1 cup wholemeal breadcrumbs, 1 dessertspoon chopped parsley, 1½ ounces butter, teaspoon salt, ¼ teaspoon pepper, 1 teaspoon chopped thyme or grated lemon rind, 1 egg.

METHOD. — Rub butter into breadcrumbs and add all other ingredients, bind with beaten egg. Place this in the prepared fish, sew up or fasten with skewer. Brush a baking dish with melted butter, lay fish on, brush over with remainder of beaten egg, and dust with browned breadcrumbs. Cover with buttered paper and cook in moderate oven about 1 hour. Test thick part of fish with skewer. Serve hot.

FISH SAVOURY

INGREDIENTS. — 1 lb. sliced uncooked fish, 1 pint wholemeal sauce, 2 tablespoons grated cheese, 1 breakfast cup wholemeal breadcrumbs, 1 teaspoon salt, ¼ teaspoon pepper, 2 teaspoons chopped parsley.

METHOD. — Place fish in a buttered casserole dish, cover with sauce, add grated cheese, sprinkle over the breadcrumbs, dot with butter and bake half an hour in moderate oven.

FISH PIE

INGREDIENTS. — 5 slices of cooked flaked fish, 2 hard boiled eggs, ½ pint sauce, 1 dessertspoon chopped parsley, seasoning, 1 breakfast cup wholemeal breadcrumbs.

METHOD. — Mix together sauce, fish, parsley and seasoning. Place in a greased pie-dish alternate layers of hard boiled eggs, fish mixture, sprinkle breadcrumbs on top, dot with butter. Bake in moderate oven.

Fruit Salads and Compotes

APPLE, ORANGE AND BANANA SALAD

INGREDIENTS. — 3 apples, 2 sweet oranges, 3 or 4 ripe bananas.

METHOD. — Peel, core and slice apples finely, quarter the oranges and slice the bananas. Pile apples in centre of dish, arrange orange round, banana on outside.

SUMMER FRUIT SALAD

INGREDIENTS. — 1 teacup red currants, ½ teacup white currants, 1 teacup gooseberry pulp.

METHOD. — Arrange white currants over gooseberry pulp, surround with red currants. Serve with whipped cream.

FIG AND APPLE SALAD

INGREDIENTS. — 4 ounces figs, 1 lb. apples, 3 tablespoons seeded raisins, cinnamon, ½ pint cream.

METHOD. — Soak figs and raisins overnight. Mince apples quickly, mix with other fruit, add cinnamon if desired, mix with cream and serve at once.

MIXED FRUIT SALAD

INGREDIENTS and METHOD. — Mix together a few stewed figs, seedless raisins, sliced or grated apple, ripe bananas and grape-fruit pulp.

SPRING FRUIT SALAD

INGREDIENTS. — 1 ripe pineapple, ½ lb. grapes, 2 juicy oranges.

WINTER FRUIT SALAD

INGREDIENTS. — 2 juicy oranges, 2 bananas, 2 large ripe apples, ½ lb. large prunes, 4 ounces walnuts, 2 egg whites, 1 tablespoon raw sugar and lemon juice.

METHOD. — Peel, core and quarter the apples, also oranges; slice bananas, chop nuts, melt sugar in lemon juice. Mix all well together. Beat whites stiffly and pile over all. Whipped cream may be used instead.

WINTER FRUIT SALAD — 2

INGREDIENTS and METHOD. — Take 1 lb. of picked dates, cook with the juice of half a lemon and a little boiling water, till they begin to swell. (Do not cook too much or dates will break up.) Pour dates and juice into dish, divide up 2 sweet oranges and arrange over dates. Allow to get quite cold. Sprinkle grated orange peel on top.

FRUIT MOUSSE

INGREDIENTS. — 1 cup of grated apple, 1 cup of mashed banana, ½ cup of chopped Brazil nuts, 2 oranges, cut fine, 1 dozen chopped dates.

DRIED FRUIT SALAD

INGREDIENTS. — 4 ounces figs, 4 ounces stoned dates, 4 ounces stoned prunes, juice of 1 lemon, 6 tablespoons of nuts, 4 ounces of Sunmaid raisins.

METHOD. — Soak prunes and figs and raisins overnight, put through mincer with other ingredients. Mix well with lemon juice, serve with cream. With the addition of a little crystallised lemon peel and currants this mixture can be used for fruit fingers if baked between wholemeal pastry.

FRUIT COMPOTE

INGREDIENTS and METHOD. — Steam some figs, prunes and dates with a little preserved ginger, with a strip of lemon peel.

FRESH FRUIT COMPOTE

INGREDIENTS and METHOD. — Use black or red currants, raspberries, etc. Crush fruit and add sufficient cereals, such as Corn flakes, to thicken. Add 1 tablespoon of grated nuts to ½ pint of fruit and sweeten with honey if necessary. Beat together and serve with cream.

FRUIT SALAD

INGREDIENTS and METHOD. — Dice 2 large bananas, 2 apples, 2 oranges, add 10 stoned dates and figs cut into small pieces, ¼ cup of raisins, and juice of 1 lemon and sugar to taste. Whipped cream and a sprinkling of chopped nuts if desired.

PEACH DELICACY

INGREDIENTS and METHOD. — Arrange a layer of sliced peaches at the bottom of the dish, and sprinkle with grated coconut, cover with layer of figs and dates chopped, then chopped pineapple and a layer of peaches to finish, sprinkled with chopped nuts and cream.

Jellies, Trifles and Cold Sweets

DATE DESSERT

INGREDIENTS and METHOD.—Wash 1 lb. of dates and simmer gently in 1 pint of milk until dates are thick and the colour of chocolate. Add juice and grated rind of 1 lemon. Cool and serve with whipped cream and decorate with nuts.

FRUIT MOULDS

INGREDIENTS and METHOD.—Equal quantities of raisins, sultanas, chopped finely, milled nuts and grated carrot. Bind to stiff paste with 2 crushed bananas and a teaspoon of honey. Press into individual moulds, turn out and serve with honey and whipped cream or custard.

ALMOND RICE MOULD

INGREDIENTS.—2 pints of milk, 4 level tablespoons brown rice, 3 drops essence of almonds, 2 ounces ground almonds, ¼ lb. raw sugar, rind of 3 a lemon.

METHOD.—Wash the rice thoroughly. Add milk, sugar, lemon peel and essence. Cook in double saucepan till dry. Add the ground almonds and cook for 6 minutes. Cool and put into glass dish. Sprinkle with ground cinnamon. Serve alone or with cream.

JELLY PLUM PUDDING

INGREDIENTS.—1 pint lemon jelly, 6 soaked prunes chopped small, 1 shredded apple, ½ cup roasted pine kernels, ¾ cup seedless raisins, grated rind of 1 orange.

METHOD.—Stir all ingredients into the lemon jelly while it is hot.

RICE CREAM

INGREDIENTS. — 2 dessertspoons Davis gelatine, 1½ cups milk, 1 cup cooked brown rice, 4 dessertspoons raw sugar, ½ cup hot water, 2 eggs, salt, vanilla.

METHOD. — Dissolve gelatine in hot water. Beat egg yolks and sugar together. Boil milk; pour gradually on to egg yolks. Place in double boiler and cook until mixture thickens. Add salt and vanilla. Leave to cool. Add gelatine, rice and stiffly whipped egg whites; pour into mould. Chopped dates or raisins may be added before the whites are stirred in.

APPLE JELLY

INGREDIENTS. — ½ lb. apples, a little ginger, 2 tablespoons brown sugar, ⅓ ounce agar or necessary amount gelatine, 1 pint water.

METHOD. — Boil apples to a pulp, cut the agar small and simmer half hour in water; add ginger. Remove ginger when agar is dissolved and add the liquid to the apple pulp. Cool, turn into mould.

APPLE DELIGHT

INGREDIENTS. — 6 apples, 1 dessertspoon honey, 3 egg whites, 1 dessertspoon gelatine, ½ pint milk, juice of 3 oranges and grated rind of two. Hot water.

METHOD. — Peel, core and grate apples. Dissolve gelatine in hot water and add to half amount of heated milk. Heat the remainder and melt honey in it, add orange rind and gradually stir in the juice. Mix together. Beat whites and mix with apples. Add the milk, etc., lightly to this. Set and use cold.

EDEN PUDDING

INGREDIENTS.—6 very ripe bananas, 1 lb. peeled and cored apples, ½ pint milk, 2 teaspoons gelatine, little honey, rind 2 lemons.

METHOD.—Simmer the cut up apples with honey and a little water. Add mashed bananas to apple when cold and mix. Prepare gelatine and lemon rind and add to the fruit.

PEACH PUDDING

INGREDIENTS and METHOD.—½ lb. simmered peaches or nectarines cut in small pieces, a little raw sugar, 4 ounces ground almonds, 1 pint milk and juice mixed, gelatine or agar agar. Mix the fruit and nuts, pour on the dissolved gelatine and juice, etc. Sprinkle with grated nutmeg when set.

PRUNE WHIP

INGREDIENTS.—1 cup cooked prunes, 3 egg whites, teaspoon vanilla essence, ¼ cup raw sugar.

METHOD.—Sieve the prunes and heat in a double boiler with the sugar 10 minutes. Remove, cool somewhat; stir in egg whites and vanilla. Serve cold with whipped cream.

APRICOT AND BOILED CUSTARD

INGREDIENTS and METHOD.—Simmer equal quantities dried soaked apricots with sweet cooking apples, washed and cut up, but not peeled or cored. When tender rub through sieve. Serve in individual glasses with custard on top and a sprinkling of chopped nuts. A little honey may be used for sweetening fruit.

MAPLE WALNUT SPONGE

INGREDIENTS.—2 cups raw sugar, ½ cup boiling water, 1¼ cups cold water, ½ cup chopped walnuts, 2 dessertspoons gelatine, pinch salt, 2 whites of eggs stiffly beaten.

METHOD.—Put sugar, salt and ¼ cup of boiling water in pan and boil for 10 minutes. Add gelatine dissolved in hot water. Stir in the cold water. When mixture begins to set whip till foamy and fold in the stiffly beaten egg whites and walnuts. Make custard with egg yolks.

BLACKBERRY FOOL

INGREDIENTS.—1 lb. blackberries, 3 tablespoons milled nuts, 4 tablespoons honey, 2 tablespoons crisped Corn flakes.

METHOD.—Crush berries and mix well with other ingredients.

FRUIT GELATINE

INGREDIENTS.—1 large dessertspoon gelatine, 1 cup hot water, 1 cup shredded apple, 2 sliced oranges, 3 sliced bananas, ½ cup nut meats.

METHOD.—Dissolve gelatine in hot water and allow to cool. When slightly thickened beat with egg beater until consistency of whipped cream. Add the fruit and nuts. Set in mould and chill.

RAISIN MAPLE BLANC-MANGE

INGREDIENTS.—1 cup seedless raisins, 3 cups boiling water, 1 cup raw sugar, a little cold water, sufficient to mix 3 small tablespoons cornflour, pinch salt, vanilla essence, a few chopped nuts.

METHOD.—Cook raisins in boiling water. Add sugar, then other ingredients and cook for 15 minutes. Serve cold.

PINEAPPLE JUNKET

INGREDIENTS.—1 pint fresh milk, 1 tablespoon sugar, 1 teaspoon rennet, few slices pineapple.

METHOD.—Heat milk till blood heat, add sugar, stir in rennet and pour into wet dish. When set put grated pineapple on top.

MOORISH PUDDING

INGREDIENTS.—4 eggs, 1 teacup milk, 2 dessertspoons gelatine, 2 tablespoons raw sugar.

METHOD.—Dissolve the gelatine in a little water (hot), heat milk over pan of boiling water and add the gelatine. Beat the egg yolks very well with the sugar, add milk and gelatine to this, then fold in the stiffly beaten egg whites flavoured with a little vanilla. Put into glass dish to set and add any kind of suitable fruit such as strawberries or raspberries when in season, quartered oranges free from pith and pips, bananas, etc., or a mixture of chopped dates, figs, ginger and crystallised cherries. Cover with whipped cream.

SPANISH CREAM

INGREDIENTS.—2 dessertspoons gelatine, 1 pint milk, 2 dessertspoons sugar, ¼ cup hot water, 2 eggs, essence of vanilla.

METHOD.—Beat yolks of eggs and sugar together; add to milk; stir over fire until mixture just comes to the boil and will coat the spoon. Remove from fire and stir in gelatine dissolved in hot water; add essence. Beat egg white until stiff and pour into mould. This mixture may be varied by lining a mould with either figs, dates or prunes. If some of the juice from these fruits is used, moderate the amount of milk or use more gelatine.

APPLE AND ALMOND CREAM

INGREDIENTS. — 5 apples, 4 ounces ground almonds, 2 ounces sugar, juice 2 lemons, 1 pint cream.

METHOD. — Whip cream with sugar. Grate apples and add lemon juice and ground almonds; leave for an hour. Then beat in lightly with the whipped cream.

Baked, Boiled or Steamed Puddings, Tarts, Custards, etc.

NOVELTY DRIED FRUIT PUDDING

INGREDIENTS.—½ cup sifted flour, ¼ cup butter, 1 teaspoon Baking Powder, 1 cup rolled oats, 1 cup raw sugar, sufficient soaked, cooked, and stoned prunes.

METHOD.—Melt butter. Add sugar, beat; add egg, and then dry ingredients. Mix well. Grease pie tin or plate and press half mixture into it. Add prunes, and cover with remainder of mixture. Bake half an hour.

HEALTH PUDDING

INGREDIENTS.—4 ounces wholemeal breadcrumbs, ¼ lb. figs, ¼ lb. raw sugar, ¼ lb. candied peel, ½ cup Golden Syrup, 4 ounces shredded suet, ¼ lb. prunes, ¼ lb. currants, 2 eggs.

METHOD.—Steam three hours. Serve with lemon sauce.

DATE AND APPLE CHARLOTTE

INGREDIENTS.—3 ounces wholemeal breadcrumbs, 1 ounce sugar, 1 beaten egg, grated rind of 1 lemon, 1 ounce butter, 2 tablespoons cream or milk, or more; 2 grated sweet apples, 1½ ounces stoned dates.

METHOD.—Mix butter, breadcrumbs, and sugar together; bind with beaten egg and milk. Add grated lemon rind and apples and dates cut into small pieces. Put in well greased dish, brush with beaten egg. Bake till nicely brown. These quantities may be used for any other dried fruit, which should be soaked overnight if necessary.

SHORT CRUST

(Good for pastries containing dates, raisins, nut mixtures, etc.)

INGREDIENTS.—1 heaped breakfast cup wholemeal flour. 1 tablespoon raw sugar, 1 egg, 1 heaped teaspoon baking powder, ¼ lb. butter.

METHOD.—Rub butter into flour and baking powder; add sugar. Mix with the eggs well beaten and a little milk.

PLAIN SHORT PASTRY

INGREDIENTS.—2 cups wholemeal flour, ½ lb. butter, milk or water to mix, ½ teaspoon baking powder, pinch salt.

METHOD.—Rub butter into flour, salt, powder, etc. Mix in enough milk to make a firm paste. Roll and fold 3 or 4 times. Bake in hot oven 10 to 15 minutes.

RICH PASTRY

INGREDIENTS.—1 cup wholemeal flour, ½ lb. butter, salt, water (about ¼ cup).

METHOD.—Mix flour and salt with water, using only enough water to make a soft paste. Roll it out. Cut up some of the butter into small pieces and roll it into the paste. Continue with butter until all is used. Set on one side in cool place for half an hour or more. Roll and fold again several times.

PLUM PUDDING

INGREDIENTS.—1 large grated apple, 2 ounces raw sugar, 2 cups Corn flakes crushed, 3 ounces butter, a little salt, nutmeg, dates, raisins, nuts, peel, etc., 1 egg, 1 dessertspoon golden syrup.

METHOD.—Prepare as usual, heating the butter and syrup before adding to dry ingredients. Steam 3 hours.

APPLE CRISP

INGREDIENTS.—4 apples, ¾ cup wholemeal flour, 2½ tablespoons butter, ½ cup sugar, ¾ cup water.

METHOD.—Slice apples into pie dish. Pour over cold water. Sprinkle with cinnamon. Rub butter into flour and sugar till crumbly, put on top of apples and bake. No sugar is required on apples as it soaks through from the crust.

RAISIN RICE

INGREDIENTS.—½ cup natural rice, 1 cup seedless raisins, 3 cups hot water.

METHOD.—Wash rice and put in casserole dish. Mix in raisins, add hot water. Cover and put in slow oven. Cook very gently till fruit is swelled and rice grains are soft. Nutmeg added when partly cooked improves the flavour.

APPLE ROLL

INGREDIENTS.—4 medium sized apples, 1 cup raw sugar, 1 pint of water.

Biscuit Dough.—2 cups wholemeal flour, 2 tablespoons sugar, 4 teaspoons baking powder, 3 tablespoons butter, ½ teaspoon salt, ½ cup milk and water.

METHOD.—Peel, core and cut fine suitable apples. Put sugar and water into deep baking pan over slow fire. While syrup is cooking slowly, make the dough. Roll out about ½ inch thick, spread with chopped apples and roll into long roll. Cut into pieces about 2 inches long, place with cut side down in the hot syrup, put small piece of butter on top, sprinkle with cinnamon and a little sugar. Bake about ¾ of an hour in moderate oven.

EVE'S PUDDING

INGREDIENTS.—2 eggs, 1 teaspoon baking powder, 4 ounces butter, 6 ounces sugar, 8 ounces wholemeal flour, little milk if necessary.

METHOD.—Cream butter and sugar, beat in eggs, add flour and milk if necessary, so that mixture resembles a sponge consistency. Pour this over prepared fruit. Apples, peaches, or stewed dried fruits may be used. Have this ready in deep pie dish and pour mixture over it. Bake in moderate oven.

FIG BRAN PUDDING

INGREDIENTS.—1 ounce of wholemeal bread broken into small pieces, 1 ounce bran, 4 ounces chopped figs, 4 ounces seeded raisins, 2 ounces chopped lemon peel, 2½ ounces butter, 1 dessertspoon sugar, 1 gill (140 ml) of milk, 1 egg.

METHOD.—Heat milk and pour on to broken bread. Cover and allow to soak ½ an hour. Beat well and add bran and sugar. Shred butter and work in with a fork. Add fruit and peel. Beat egg and bind mixture. Put in greased basin and steam 3 hours or longer; or bake in very slow oven for 1½ hours. Other dried fruit may be used instead of figs.

FAVOURITE PUDDING

INGREDIENTS.—2 lb. juicy red cooking apples, 2 tablespoons of raisins, 1 tablespoon sugar, milled nuts, 2 tablespoons of grated lemon or orange peel.

METHOD.—Wash apples and grate with skin. Add sugar, soaked raisins, peel and mix. Sprinkle liberally with nuts. Place casserole or baking dish in moderate oven and bake till quite hot, but only slightly brown.

PRUNE DELICACY

INGREDIENTS.—1 lb. prunes, 2 grated apples, 1 tablespoon raw sugar, white 1 egg.

METHOD.—Soak and cook prunes, mash well with grated apple and sugar. Well whip egg white and add very gradually. Bake for a few minutes to brown.

RHUBARB GRANOSE

INGREDIENTS and METHOD.—Butter a pie-dish thickly and sprinkle with sugar and coat with a thick layer of Corn flakes. Put in a good layer of stewed sweetened rhubarb, cover with more Corn flakes and sugar. Dot with butter and bake for 20 minutes.

DATE SOUFFLÉ

INGREDIENTS.—¾ lb. dates or ½ lb. stoned dates, 1 cup water, 1 tablespoon lemon juice, 3 egg whites.

METHOD.—Cover stoned dates with water and stand 5 hours. Then cook slowly in some of the water and rub through coarse sieve. Add lemon juice and stir in stiffly beaten egg whites. Pour into a buttered dish and stand in a pan of.hot water and bake till firm. May be eaten either hot or cold.

RAISIN PUDDING

INGREDIENTS and METHOD.—Soak one cup of wholemeal breadcrumbs in water. Beat up with fork and add 1 cup raisins, ½ cup bran, 1 tablespoon raw sugar, a little spice or nutmeg. Steam in buttered basin about 2 hours or bake in slow oven 1 hour.

DATE AND FIG PIE WITH CHOCOLATE SAUCE

INGREDIENTS.—½ lb. stoned dates, 2 tablespoons flour, 1 teaspoon baking powder, ½ lb. figs, 1 ounce sugar, 1 egg, 1 cup wholemeal breadcrumbs, 1 cup milk, 3 ounces butter.

METHOD.—Stew figs till tender (first soaking overnight) in as little water as possible, drain and take out; then cut up in small pieces. Chop the dates, rub the butter into the flour and breadcrumbs, add baking powder, sugar, figs and dates. Beat egg in milk and add to mixture. Beat all well. Put in well greased dish and bake about hour. Serve with sauce.

Sauce: ½ pint milk, 1 egg yoke, small dessertspoon cocoa, sugar to taste, vanilla. Beat yolk of egg well with sugar. Boil milk with cocoa and pour over the egg yolk. Stir over slow fire until it thickens. Add essence and serve.

COTTAGE PUDDING

INGREDIENTS.—1 quart milk, 1 tablespoon sugar, grated lemon rind, 1 pint wholemeal breadcrumbs, 4 egg yolks, 1 large tablespoon butter.

METHOD.—Mix and bake till set. Beat a small cup sugar and juice of lemon together and spread over pudding. Beat egg whites and pile on top. Lightly brown in oven.

APPLE GOODY

INGREDIENTS and METHOD.—Slice ripe apples to fill a deep buttered dish; squeeze over them the juice of a large orange and grate over some of the peel. To a quart of apple add cup raw sugar. Mix lightly, dot with butter and bake till rich and soft but not too dry; when nearly finished sprinkle with chopped almonds. Eat either cold or hot, preferably cold.

PRUNE, APRICOT OR APPLE BETTY

INGREDIENTS and METHOD. — Cover the bottom of a buttered dish with coarse wholemeal breadcrumbs. Add a layer of cooked stewed prunes (or other fruit), dust with cinnamon, nutmeg and raw sugar. Fill dish with these layers, finishing with breadcrumbs. Cover with hot milk and bake 30 minutes.

PRUNE ROLL

INGREDIENTS. — ½ lb. soaked prunes, 1 dessertspoon raw sugar, 3 ounces each wholemeal flour, chopped candied peel, wholemeal breadcrumbs.

METHOD. — Mix all together and bake in buttered dish 1 hour in moderate oven.

APPLE PUFF

INGREDIENTS and METHOD. — Two cups peeled grated apples. Beat 4 egg whites and sweeten. Stir into apples with the juice of 1 lemon. Bake for 25 minutes, moderate oven. Use egg yolks for custard and serve with it.

CARROT PUDDING

INGREDIENTS. — ¼ lb. carrots, ¾ lb. wholemeal breadcrumbs, ¼ lb. butter, 1 egg, 2 ounces each raw sugar and cherries, ½ teaspoon cinnamon.

METHOD. — Put cooked carrots through sieve. Cream butter and sugar. Beat egg white stiff. Add crumbs, carrot, yolk, cinnamon and cherries to butter and sugar. Mix in egg white and steam 2½ hours in buttered basin.

FIG PUDDING

INGREDIENTS.—½ lb. figs, 2 ounces butter, ½ lb. wholemeal bread, ¾ pint milk, 2 eggs.

METHOD.—Soak figs in hot water 24 hours. Stew in same water till tender, then cut into small pieces. Dice bread. Warm milk and butter and mix well, and pour over the bread. Stand for 10 minutes and then mix in the figs and lemon juice. Beat eggs, add and steam 3 hours.

POTATO PUDDING

INGREDIENTS.—3 cooked potatoes, 2 ounces ground almonds, 3 eggs, ½ lb. raw sugar, ½ teacup wholemeal breadcrumbs, grated rind and juice of a lemon.

METHOD.—Mash potatoes and add almonds, sugar, breadcrumbs and then rind and juice. Beat eggs thoroughly and add. Mix and stand for ¼ hour. Bake or steam 1 hour.

FIG AND RAISIN PUDDING

INGREDIENTS.—½ lb. chopped figs, ¼ lb. chopped raisins, ½ lb. breadcrumbs, 1 egg, milk, vanilla.

METHOD.—Stir all together to make a rather damp mixture. Let stand 1 hour. Put into well buttered mould and steam 2 hours. Turn out carefully, serve with sauce.

PRUNE AND FIG SHAPE

INGREDIENTS and METHOD.—Line a buttered basin with soaked stoned prunes or figs split in half, seeded side to mould. Soak 2 ounces stale breadcrumbs in ½ pint milk. Add 4 ounces raw sugar and 2 beaten eggs. Add this carefully to mould. Tie over buttered paper and steam 1 hour.

RAISIN OR SULTANA PUDDING

INGREDIENTS. — ¼ lb. each wholemeal flour, butter and breadcrumbs, 1 egg, ½ lb. seeded raisins, 1 tablespoon raw sugar, mixed peel to taste.

METHOD. — Work butter into flour and crumbs, add fruit, etc., and egg last, also a little milk. Steam 2 hours.

PATRICIA PUDDING

INGREDIENTS. — ½ lb. grated carrots, ½ lb. Corn flakes, ¼ lb. currants, ½ nutmeg, teaspoon ground cloves, apple, banana, yolk of egg and a little prune juice.

METHOD. — Mix dry ingredients and bind with prune juice to which has been added a few drops lemon juice and beaten egg yolk. Steam 3 hours.

STEAMED DATE PUDDING

INGREDIENTS and METHOD. — Four ounces wholemeal pastry, 6 ounces chopped dates, grated lemon rind and juice. Line a basin with pastry, fill with date mixture, top with pastry and steam 2½ hours.

STEAMED CHOCOLATE PUDDING

INGREDIENTS. — 3 ounces sugar, 5 ounces of wheaten breadcrumbs, ¾ pint of milk, ¼ lb. of Mexican chocolate, 3 yolks, 3 whites of eggs, vanilla flavouring.

METHOD. — Grate chocolate and dissolve in milk with sugar. Put bread crumbs into basin and pour chocolate mixture over. Add beaten up yolks. Whisk whites stiffly and stir in lightly. Turn into buttered mould and steam 1 hour.

SPANISH PUDDING

INGREDIENTS.—3 ounces sultanas, 2 ounces of ground almonds, 2 ounces of butter, 2 ounces of citron peel, 4 ounces of breadcrumbs, 3 eggs.

METHOD.—Melt butter and mix with breadcrumbs, add ground almonds, sultanas, chopped peel, and eggs well beaten. Use a little milk if necessary. Steam 40 to 60 minutes.

STEAMED TREACLE SPONGE

INGREDIENTS.—½ lb. of butter, ½ lb. of treacle, ½ lb. of wholemeal flour, ¼ lb. of sugar, ½ pint of milk, 2 eggs.

METHOD.—Beat butter and sugar to a cream, add eggs and beat for 20 minutes. Add milk and treacle and lastly flour, put in a greased basin and steam 1½ hours.

STEAMED TREACLE PUDDING

INGREDIENTS.—6 ounces of wholemeal flour, 3 ounces of butter, ½ a gill (70 ml) of water, treacle.

METHOD.—Rub butter into flour with finger tips, make into stiff dough, roll out on to board and cut into 4 or 5 pieces. Line greased basin with 1 large piece of pastry, and put treacle in bottom, then another piece of pastry, more treacle, and so on till basin is full. Cover with greased paper and then tie over a cloth. Steam 1½ to 2 hours.

STUFFED PEARS OR APPLES

INGREDIENTS and METHOD.—Core large fruits, stuff with nuts, raisins, dates, etc., and sweeten with honey and bake.

CANARY PUDDING

INGREDIENTS.—6 ripe bananas, 3 ounces Corn Flakes, 1 egg, ½ pint of milk, 4 ounces of sultanas.

METHOD.—Beat egg thoroughly and add it to the milk, adding a little sugar if desired. Pour this over the Corn flakes and sultanas, and let them soak for ½ hour. Mash the bananas and add to mixture. Pour into greased dish and bake 30 to 40 minutes until just brown. Oven not very hot.

ALMOND AND RAISIN TART

INGREDIENTS.—4 ounces seedless raisins, 2 ounces ground almonds, 1 ounce raw sugar, 1 egg white, 1 dessertspoon orange juice, a few whole almonds, wholemeal pastry.

METHOD.—Line a shallow dish or tin with pastry. Put raisins in (they should be soaked overnight and the water strained off), mix ground almonds with orange juice and sugar and water from the raisins, stir in beaten white, spread lightly over the raisins and decorate with blanched almonds. Bake about 1½ hours in moderate oven.

FIG ROLL

INGREDIENTS.—1 breakfast cup each Corn flakes and wholemeal flour, 3 ounces butter, 2 ounces finely grated coconut, ¾ lb. chopped figs, some sweet grated apple.

METHOD.—Mix flour, Corn flakes and coconut; work in butter, mix to a stiff paste with water and roll out into a long thin strip. Damp all over and spread the chopped figs evenly, then sprinkle raw grated apple over, wet edges and roll over. Put 2 pieces of grease-proof paper or tie in cloth. Steam 2½ hours or bake ¾ hour.

SWEET WHOLEMEAL PASTRY

INGREDIENTS. — 3 ounces butter, 2 tablespoons sugar, egg, heaped breakfast cup wholemeal flour, 1 teaspoon cream tartar, ½ teaspoon baking soda.

METHOD. — Cream butter and sugar, add beaten egg, mix cream of tartar and soda with flour and add to mixture (this may be used occasionally for mince pies, apple or dried fruit shortcake, marmalade tarts, etc.).

WHOLEMEAL PASTRY — 1

INGREDIENTS. — 4 ounces wholemeal flour, 2 ounces butter, 1 ounce Soyolk (soya flour), ½ gill (70ml) water, lemon juice.

METHOD. — Put flour on board and add Soyolk and chop in butter with a knife. Lift the flour a good deal and chop lightly. Mix a few drops of lemon juice with the water. Chop water in also, just a little at a time and hardly touch with hands. Roll out in small quantities at a time, roll away from you and do not fold.

WHOLEMEAL PASTRY — 2

INGREDIENTS. — 1½ cups wholemeal flour, ½ cup water, ¼ lb. butter.

METHOD. — Shave butter into flour, mix with water and roll out ready for use.

DATE OR FIG CUSTARD

INGREDIENTS and METHOD. — Well butter a dish and press halved stoned dates or cooked figs to bottom and sides so that whole dish is well covered. Pour in custard and bake in pan of water in moderate oven.

BANANAS IN LEMON SYRUP

INGREDIENTS and METHOD.—Skin about ½ dozen bananas and either slice them or leave whole. Make a syrup of 1 large cup of water and 1½ cups raw sugar, boil until reduced to half this quantity. Add the grated rind of a lemon and the juice (do not boil these or the syrup will be bitter), pour very hot over the bananas and cover. Serve cold with cream.

BANANA FLAKES

INGREDIENTS and METHOD.—Peel as many bananas as wanted and lay in flat dish. Pour over the juice of 1 or 2 oranges sweetened with raw sugar. Let these soak for an hour or longer. Lift from dish and drain. Beat up an egg, roll bananas in this, then roll thoroughly in Corn flakes. Dip in egg once more and fry until crisp and brown. (These may be baked in oven until crisp if preferred.) The orange juice left over after bananas have been soaked may be used for sauce.

BAKED BANANAS

INGREDIENTS and METHOD.—Peel bananas, lie side by side it a shallow dish, which has been well buttered and covered with sugar. Sprinkle more sugar over bananas, and squeeze juice of 1 lemon. Add a little water, cover and bake 20 minutes.

PRUNE MERINGUE

INGREDIENTS and METHOD.—Cook gently 1 lb. of prunes, remove stones and chop up. Add juice of half a lemon, and a large cup full of breadcrumbs. Butter pie-dish and fill it with alternate layers of prunes and breadcrumbs. Pour over half pint of custard, put whipped white of egg on top. Bake 20 minutes.

GOLDEN CUSTARD

INGREDIENTS.—3 eggs, 1 pint of milk, 3 tablespoons of cream, 1 good teaspoon of honey.

METHOD.—Warm milk and dissolve honey in it. Whisk eggs and pour in milk. Stand basin in hot water over slow gas, stir until creamy. Remove from fire, add a few drops of essence and add cream, letting it cool a little first. Put a thick layer of lemon or orange curd in fancy dish, pour over custard and decorate.

Fruit Sauces, etc. and Fillings for Tarts and Cakes

LEMON CURD

INGREDIENTS.—1 lb. thick honey, 4 large eggs or 3 duck eggs, 3 ounces butter, juice of 3 large lemons, grated rind of 1 or 2 oranges.

METHOD.—Beat honey and work in butter. Beat eggs and thoroughly mix into honey and butter. Add grated rinds and lemon juice and beat again. Cook in double boiler until it thickens. Keep in covered jars.

SWISS JELLY

INGREDIENTS.—2 eggs, 3 gills (420 ml) milk, 1 tablespoon honey, vanilla essence, nuts, 1½ dessertspoons gelatine, a little hot water.

METHOD.—Dissolve gelatine in water and add to the heated milk. Add honey and vanilla and cool. Then add well beaten egg yolks, and stir well. Set. Use in small tartlets with egg whites sweetened and set in meringue.

MUSCAT JELLY

INGREDIENTS.—1 dessertspoon raw sugar, ½ packet seeded raisins, strained juice 1 lemon, 2 dessertspoons gelatine.

METHOD.—Soak raisins over night. Strain off liquor and make up to 1 pint. Add the gelatine previously dissolved in a little hot water and cook very gently for 20 minutes. Put soaked raisins in dish and pour over liquid and lemon juice. Allow to cool.

BANANA MINCEMEAT

INGREDIENTS.—½ lb. skinned bananas, ½ lb. soft candied peel, ¼ lb. seeded raisins, ¼ lb. raw sugar, 1 ounce almonds, ¼ grated nutmeg, ½ lemon rind and juice, ¼ lb. each currants, sultanas, peeled apples, a little almond essence.

METHOD.—Chop the peel, fruit and nuts and mix with the bananas and essence. Tie in air-tight jar, when it will keep indefinitely.

FRUIT SAUCE

INGREDIENTS and METHOD.—Simmer together lemon and orange rind, also the pairings of apples. Strain and thicken with a little cornflour.

RAISIN SAUCE

INGREDIENTS and METHOD.—Mix wholemeal flour, sugar and butter into paste with milk and cook to a creamy consistency. Press 1 ounce soaked cooked raisins through a sieve and add.

LEMON SAUCE

INGREDIENTS and METHOD.—Cream ½ cup butter and 1 heaped cup raw sugar, add grated rind of a lemon and 4 tablespoons lemon juice. Beat thoroughly and cook for a few moments over low heat, stirring all the time.

PRUNE AND APPLE SAUCE

INGREDIENTS and METHOD.—Stone and mash cooked prunes through a sieve. Grate 1 pound sweet apples. Steam together about 10 minutes with a little raw sugar.

BERRY SAUCE

INGREDIENTS and METHOD.—2 cups berries (strawberries, raspberries, loganberries, etc.). Steam in a little water until tender; add raw sugar.

RAW BERRY SAUCE

Crush berries and sweeten with honey or raw sugar. Do not cook.

HONEY SAUCE

INGREDIENTS and METHOD.—One-third cupful whipped cream to half cup honey. Add the melted honey slowly to whipped cream, beating constantly.

ORANGE CURD

Proceed as for lemon curd substituting 2 oranges and 1 lemon.

HOME CANDIED PEEL

INGREDIENTS.—Peel of 6 tangerines, 3 tablespoons honey, ½ breakfast cup hot water.

METHOD.—Melt honey in hot water in small jar, add peel and cook gently until soft and syrupy. Turn out of jar to cool, then cover and keep till needed. If this natural conserve is cut into thin strips and used in any wholemeal cakes or puddings it gives a delicious flavour to them. The peel of ordinary lemons or oranges can also be utilised in the same way, but it is first necessary to cook the peel in a little water and scrape out the pith. Then proceed as above. Lemon and grapefruit need rather more honey.

FRUIT FILLING—1

INGREDIENTS.—1 tablespoon wholemeal flour, ½ breakfast cup water, 2 ounces raw sugar, ½ lemon rind and juice, ½ cup each seeded raisins and chopped walnuts.

METHOD.—Boil sugar and water. Mix flour and lemon juice and add to liquid. Stir till it boils and boil 3 minutes. Add minced fruit and nuts. Cool and use between pastry or cake.

FRUIT FILLING—2

INGREDIENTS and METHOD.—Half packet seeded raisins, 2 ounces almonds. Put through mincer and mix in 1 tablespoon lemon juice.

FRUIT FILLING—3

As above, but using dates and walnuts instead of other ingredients.

FRUIT FILLING—4

INGREDIENTS and METHOD.—Half cup each chopped figs, dates, raisins, nuts and preserved ginger, 3 tablespoons each lemon juice and boiling water, 1 tablespoon sugar. Mix ingredients, cook in double saucepan till thick. Use warm.

RAISIN CREAM FILLING

INGREDIENTS.—½ cup cream stiffly beaten, ½ cup seeded raisins and 2 tablespoons nuts put through mincer, ½ teaspoon gelatine dissolved in 2 tablespoons milk, 1 ounce castor sugar.

METHOD.—Soak gelatine in milk for 5 minutes. Heat gently. Cool and add to other ingredients. Mix well and use before it becomes too set.

RAISIN CARAMEL FROSTING

INGREDIENTS. — 1 cup raw sugar, ¼ cup water, 1 stiffly beaten egg white, ¾ cup raisins, vanilla essence.

METHOD. — Cook sugar and water 5 minutes. Remove and when bubbling ceases stir in egg white. Beat till thick enough to spread. Add raisins.

Wholemeal Breads, Scones, Loaves, Slices

TREACLE BREAD

INGREDIENTS.—1 lb. wholemeal flour, 6 ounces butter, 1 heaped teaspoon caraway seeds, ½ teaspoon mixed spice, 1 teacup black treacle, about 1 gill (140 ml) sour milk.

METHOD.—Mix flour, caraway seeds and spice. Rub in butter, warm the treacle by standing in hot water for a little while; mix into other ingredients; add milk last. Make rather on the wet side but not too moist. Bake 45 to 60 minutes in a well greased rather shallow tin.

WHOLEMEAL BREAD

INGREDIENTS.—2 cups flour, 2 teaspoons yeast, 1 teaspoon sugar, little salt, less than 1 teacup tepid water.

METHOD.—Cream yeast and sugar, add water. Make a well in the middle of the warmed flour, pour in liquid and mix with wooden spoon. Beat well. Turn on to floured board and knead lightly. Place in greased tins and allow loaves to rise till double their original size. Bake 30 minutes in hot oven.

EXCELLENT WHOLEMEAL BREAD

INGREDIENTS.—4 cups flour, 8 teaspoons Soyolk (soya flour), ¼ ounce compressed yeast, 1 or 2 teaspoons raw sugar, 1 teaspoon salt, 2 cups warm water.

METHOD.—Mix the yeast and sugar, add warm water and pour into the warmed flour. Leave 10 minutes. Mix, set and then knead in the usual way. Set only once.

FAMILY WHOLEMEAL BREAD

INGREDIENTS and METHOD.—Mix ¾ ounce compressed yeast with 1 tablespoon raw sugar, and when creamy add 1 cupful of lukewarm water. Heat another cup of water and mix in it 1 or 2 tablespoons treacle. Add this to 1 pint of potato water (without salt) and mix yeast, etc., to this, making sure the liquid is only luke warm, otherwise heat will kill the yeast. Sift in 2 cups white flour and make into a batter with the liquid; using a warmed basin. To this stir in 1 cup of bran and 7 cups wholemeal flour which has been warmed and 1 tablespoon salt added to it. Knead lightly and leave to rise for 4 or 5 hours. Divide and knead again. Put into greased tins and leave another ½ hour in warm place. Bake in a good oven 1 hour.

WHOLEMEAL SCONES

INGREDIENTS.—3 cups wholemeal flour, 1 teaspoon baking soda, 1 tablespoon butter, 2 teaspoons cream of tartar.

METHOD.—Heat the butter, but do not make it runny and rub into the flour. Mix all with 2 tablespoons melted treacle and enough milk to make into a soft dough. Roll out and bake 15 to 25 minutes.

POTATO SCONES

INGREDIENTS and METHOD.—Pass a cupful of cooked boiled potatoes through a sieve and warm in saucepan with 2 tablespoons raw sugar, and 1 tablespoon butter until smooth and creamy. Beat an egg and add to potato mixture, and stir in a salt-spoon of salt and 2 cupfuls of wheatmeal flour into which has been sifted 1½ teaspoons baking powder. Work to a smooth scone consistency with a little milk. Roll out and bake in fairly hot oven.

PUMPKIN SCONES

Same quantities and method as for Potato Scones.

BRAN SCONES

INGREDIENTS.—3 cups bran, ¼ lb. butter, 1 cup fine wholemeal, raisins if liked, 1 cup coarse wholemeal.

METHOD.—Rub butter into dry ingredients, sift in 2 teaspoons baking powder, beat up 1 egg in a breakfast cup of milk. Roll out and bake in low oven for 1 hour.

SPICE SCONES

INGREDIENTS.—½ lb. wholemeal, 1 ounce butter, 1 tablespoon golden syrup, 1 tablespoon raw sugar, I teaspoon each bicarbonate of soda, ground cinnamon, mixed spice, pinch of salt, sour milk to mix.

METHOD.—Rub butter into flour, add sugar, spices, soda and salt. Mix thoroughly. Add to the syrup and use sufficient sour milk or buttermilk, about 1 gill (140ml), to mix into a light dough. Roll out ½ inch thick and bake in a hot scone oven.

WHOLEMEAL FRUIT LOAF

INGREDIENTS.—1 lb. wholemeal flour, ¼ lb. each sultanas and currants, 5 ounces raw sugar, 2 ounces butter, 2 teaspoons baking powder, ½ to 1 teaspoon mixed spice according to taste.

METHOD.—Beat butter and sugar to a cream, stir in other ingredients, and add about ½ breakfast cupful cold water or milk. A little more liquid if the mixture seems too stiff. Form into flat loaf, coat with flour, and bake 1¼ hours on baking slide.

RAISIN SCONES

INGREDIENTS.—3 cups wholemeal flour, 1 ounce butter, a little salt, 1¾ cups milk, 1 cup seeded raisins, 2 teaspoons baking powder.

METHOD.—Rub butter into flour, add raisins, then milk to make a soft dough. Brush over with milk and bake in hot oven.

LOVE KNOTS

INGREDIENTS and METHOD.—To 1 lb. wholemeal flour rub in a little butter, add 1 cup sour cream (thick). Roll out, cut into strips and fold like figure 8. Bake in moderate oven.

OATMEAL SLICES

INGREDIENTS and METHOD.—Make some thick porridge of coarse oatmeal. Turn into a flat dish and cover to prevent a crust forming. When cold and required for use, cut into slices less than 1 inch thick, pass through seasoned flour, then egg and breadcrumbs. Fry a golden brown in boiling fat, and serve piping hot. These slices may be made more savoury by the addition of a little finely grated onion, a salt-spoon or more of dried herbs, and a little pepper and salt added while the porridge is being cooked.

MUSCATEL BREAD

INGREDIENTS.—½ pint milk, sour or sweet, 1 lb. wholemeal flour, 6 ounces butter, 1 packet seeded raisins.

METHOD.—Rub butter into flour lightly, add raisins and mix to a moderately stiff paste with milk. Cook 15 minutes in a greased shallow tin (uncovered), then cover with another tin and cook in a fairly swift oven 40 minutes. Very good eaten with nut butter.

WHOLEMEAL HONEY SCONES

INGREDIENTS.—2 cups wholemeal flour, 1 cup white flour, 1 tablespoon butter, 2 tablespoons honey, 1 egg, ½ cup chopped dates, 2 teaspoons baking powder.

METHOD.—Rub butter into flour, add other ingredients, then make a soft dough. Brush over with milk and bake in hot oven.

WHOLEMEAL NUT LOAF

INGREDIENTS.—3 cups wholemeal flour, 2 tablespoons butter, a little salt, 1 small teaspoon baking powder, 2 cups sultanas, 1 large cup chopped nuts, 1 tablespoon raw sugar, enough milk to make a stiffish dough.

METHOD.—Rub butter into dry ingredients, and mix together with as little milk as will make a very stiff dough. Press into a greased tin and bake slowly for 1 hour. The loaf should turn out very solid. Do not cut until quite cold.

NUT AND DATE LOAF

INGREDIENTS.—2 cups wholemeal flour, 1 cup each chopped dates, walnuts and milk, 1 egg, 2 teaspoons baking powder, ½ teaspoon salt.

METHOD.—Mix all dry ingredients; add egg and milk. Bake in tin 1 hour.

BRAN MUFFINS

INGREDIENTS.—1 teacup each wholemeal flour, golden syrup and milk, 2 teacups bran, 1 level teaspoon baking soda dissolved in milk, ½ teaspoon baking powder.

METHOD.—Mix well and half fill greased patty pans; bake moderate oven about 15 minutes.

CURRANT BREAD

INGREDIENTS. — ½ lb. wholemeal flour, 2 ounces butter, 6 ounces currants, 1½ ounces raw sugar, 1 teaspoon baking powder, pinch of salt, milk.

METHOD. — Mix dry ingredients, rub in butter. Mix to stiff dough with milk. Knead into a light round loaf, place in well greased tin and bake in hot oven ¾ hour, reducing heat after 20 minutes.

OATCAKES

INGREDIENTS. — 6 ounces coarse oatmeal, ½ teacup raw sugar, 6 ounces fine wholemeal flour, ¼ lb. butter, milk to mix.

METHOD. — Rub butter into wholemeal flour and oatmeal, add sugar, stir well. Mix to a very stiff dough with a little milk. Roll out thinly, cut into squares, and bake in a moderate-hot oven till slightly browned.

RUSKS

INGREDIENTS. — 2 breakfast cups wholemeal flour, 2 small tablespoons butter, 1 ounce raw sugar, 1 egg, milk to mix.

METHOD. — Rub butter lightly into flour; add sugar, beaten egg and mix with milk. Knead lightly, roll ¼-inch thick and cut. Bake in a quick oven until risen but not brown. Split open, return to oven (cool) until golden brown and crisp.

Biscuits: Plain, Savoury and Sweet

ROLLED OAT BISCUITS

INGREDIENTS.—3 cups rolled oats, 1½ cups wholemeal flour, ¼ lb. butter, 3 tablespoons syrup, 1 egg.

METHOD.—Work together butter, syrup and egg; add oats and flour. Roll out, cut in suitable shape and bake in moderate oven.

PLAIN WHOLEMEAL BISCUITS

INGREDIENTS.—4 ounces butter, 1 cup milk, 1 egg, 12 ounces wholemeal flour, 1 teaspoon lemon juice.

METHOD.—Rub butter into flour, add egg and lemon juice and enough milk to make a stiff paste. Roll out thin and bake in moderate oven.

SAVOURY CHEESE BISCUITS

INGREDIENTS.—1 teacup wholemeal flour, 4 ounces grated cheese, 2 ounces butter, 1 teaspoon Marmite.

METHOD.—Rub butter into flour, add cheese. Dissolve Marmite in a little warm milk and water; stir into mixture but keep rather dry. Roll out thinly, cut in small rounds, prick well and bake in sharp oven.

WHOLEMEAL CHEESE STRAWS

INGREDIENTS.—2 ounces wholemeal flour, 2 ounces grated cheese, 1½ ounces butter, a small egg.

METHOD.—Mix flour, cheese and butter; add beaten egg. Roll out in thin strips, and bake in very moderate oven 8 to 10 minutes.

CHEESE AND POTATO BISCUITS

INGREDIENTS. — ½ lb. freshly mashed potatoes, ¼ lb. wholemeal flour, ¼ lb. fine oatmeal, ¼ lb. butter, 3 ounces grated cheese, ½ to 1 teaspoon celery salt.

METHOD. — Mix all dry ingredients; beat in the potato. Melt butter and work in. Mix to a paste with milk (sour preferred). Roll out on well floured board. Cut, dip in medium oatmeal and bake on well greased tins 15 to 20 minutes in a sharp oven. Eat with salad or vegetable stew.

LUNCHIES

INGREDIENTS. — 1 cup wholemeal flour, ½ teaspoon ginger, ½ cup raw sugar, 1 cup coconut, 1 teaspoon baking powder, 1 egg, ½ teaspoon cinnamon, 4 ounces butter.

METHOD. — Rub butter into wholemeal flour, add all dry ingredients, mix in beaten egg, roll out thinly, cut into squares. Bake in moderate oven.

NUT BISCUITS

INGREDIENTS. — 1 large cup wholemeal flour, 1 egg, 1 cup chopped nuts, ¼ lb. butter, 1 cup raw sugar.

METHOD. — Cream the butter and sugar; add egg well beaten; then the flour; a little essence of vanilla and the nuts. Break off pieces; put on a greased slide and bake slowly till golden brown.

FRUIT BISCUITS

INGREDIENTS. — 1 cup coconut, ½ cup walnuts, ½ cup dates, ½ cup seeded raisins, 1 cup figs, 1 small tin condensed milk.

METHOD. — Chop fruit and nuts, add coconut and mix well. Bind with milk. Put in spoonfuls on cold tray and cook in slow oven.

THREE-A-PENNY BISCUITS

INGREDIENTS. — ½ lb. wholemeal, ¼ lb. sugar, ¼ lb. butter, small ½ cup new milk, vanilla, pinch salt.

METHOD. — Rub butter into meal, sugar and salt. Add vanilla and milk. Roll out thin, cut into shapes and bake in medium oven about 10 minutes.

LEMON RINGS

INGREDIENTS. — ¾ lb. wholemeal flour, ¼ lb. each butter and sugar, ½ gill (70ml) milk, 2 eggs, grated rind 2 lemons, a little lemon essence.

METHOD. — Cream butter and sugar; add well beaten eggs, milk, flour, rind, etc. Roll out ¼-inch thick, cut with round cutter stamped with a small round inside. Bake in moderate oven.

SPONGE BISCUITS

INGREDIENTS. — 1 cup sugar, 3 eggs, ¼ lb. butter, 1½ cups wholemeal flour, 1 teaspoon baking powder, a little lemon honey (any filling will do such as cream or minced dates, etc.).

METHOD. — Beat butter and sugar to a cream; add egg yolks and beat well. Stir in baking powder and flour, and lastly egg whites beaten stiff. Put in half teaspoonfuls on a cold slide and bake in hot oven about 5 minutes. Put together with the desired filling.

GOLDEN SYRUP BISCUITS

INGREDIENTS. — ½ lb. wholemeal flour, ½ teaspoon baking powder, 2 tablespoons golden syrup, 4 ounces butter, 2 ounces sugar, pinch salt.

METHOD. — Cream butter, sugar and golden syrup. Stir in flour, salt and baking powder. Knead well and bake in a moderate oven about 15 minutes.

BUTTER BISCUITS

INGREDIENTS.—½ lb. each butter and wholemeal flour, 3 ounces raw sugar, ½ ounce cinnamon, a little ground ginger and spice, 1 egg.

METHOD.—Cream butter and sugar, add well beaten egg and dry ingredients. Roll out very thin, decorate top with sliced peel, and bake in moderate oven.

HONEY BISCUITS

INGREDIENTS.—4 ounces honey, 8 ounces butter, ¾ lb. wholemeal flour, 1 egg, grated rind 2 oranges.

METHOD.—Beat butter and honey to a cream; add orange rind and flour. Mix with egg (but do not use this if mixture already seems thin); roll out quickly and cut into squares. Put on floured trays and bake slowly 20 to 30 minutes.

LUNCH SQUARES

INGREDIENTS.—8 ounces wholemeal our, 6 ounces butter, 3 ounces honey.

METHOD.—Cream butter and honey; add flour. Roll out on grease-proof paper, cut in two. Spread one half with following mixture: 1 cup raisins, a little grated lemon or orange peel, 1 tablespoon raw sugar, 2 tablespoons warm milk, and a little melted butter. Add just sufficient wholemeal breadcrumbs to firm the mixture. Flavour with cinnamon, cover with the other half pastry and bake 20 to 30 minutes in moderate oven. Cut into squares when cold.

DATE CRACKERS

INGREDIENTS and METHOD. — Cook 1 lb. dates with cup cold water until dates are soft. Allow to cool and spread between layers of the following mixture: 2½ cups wholemeal flour, 2½ cups rolled oats, 1 cup butter, small cup raw sugar, ½ cup hot water. Rub butter in lightly; add other ingredients and mix well. Roll out thin in rolled oats, spread with date mixture and cover with same. Cut into squares and bake.

BRAN BISCUITS

INGREDIENTS. — 3 cups of bran, 1 cup of wholemeal flour, 4 ounces of butter, ½ cup of brown sugar, 2 teaspoons of baking powder, 1 egg, milk to mix.

METHOD. — Beat butter and sugar to a cream, add egg and milk to make a stiff dough, roll out thin. Bake till brown, about ¼ hour. Eggs may be omitted.

Fruit, Sponge, and Small Cakes

SULTANA LUNCH CAKE

INGREDIENTS.—3 ounces each butter and sugar, 1 egg, ¾ teacup milk, ½ lb. wholemeal flour, nutmeg, 1 ounce grated lemon peel, 1 teacup sultanas.

METHOD.—Cream butter and sugar; add well beaten egg, flour and fruit. Cook in shallow greased tin in good oven 40 minutes.

GINGER BRAN CAKE

INGREDIENTS.—½ lb. wholemeal flour, 3 ounces bran, 1 ounce raw sugar, 1 egg, 1 teaspoon each ground ginger, mixed spice, 4 ounces butter, 6 ounces seedless raisins, 1 small teacup black treacle, 2 tablespoons thick sour milk, 4 ounces lemon peel, 2 ounces chopped ginger.

METHOD.—Mix flour, ginger, spice and sugar thoroughly; add raisins and peel. Warm treacle (not hot) and add sour milk to it; then add the beaten egg. Warm butter and add first to dry goods, then the treacle, egg, milk. Mix well, pour into shallow tin and bake in slow oven 1¼ to 1½ hours. Leave in tin until cold.

PEACE CAKE

INGREDIENTS.—2 cups raw sugar, 2 tablespoons butter, 1 teaspoon cinnamon, 2 cups hot water, 1 teaspoon clove, 1 packet seeded raisins.

METHOD.—Boil all together for 5 minutes after it bubbles. When cool, add 1 teaspoon soda dissolved in 1 tablespoon hot water, and 3 cups flour, bake in moderate oven 45 minutes.

BRAN PARKINS

INGREDIENTS.—4 ounces oatmeal, 2 ounces bran, 1 ounce wholemeal flour, 4 ounces butter, 1 egg, 1 teacup black treacle, 4 ounces seedless raisins, 2 ounces chopped mixed peel, ¼ teaspoon each cinnamon, mixed spice and ground ginger, 1 ounce raw sugar.

METHOD.—Mix oatmeal, bran, wholemeal flour, sugar, peel and fruit. Warm butter and treacle (not too hot), add beaten egg to them, and work into dry ingredients. Bake in shallow greased tin 1½ hours in very slow oven. Turn off oven and leave another half hour.

WHOLEMEAL WALNUT CAKE

INGREDIENTS.—2 ounces butter, 2 ounces Soyolk (soya flour), 2 ounces wholemeal flour, 2 ounces raw sugar, 2 eggs, 6 ounces milled walnuts, 2 ounces chopped walnuts, 1 egg to bind chopped walnuts.

METHOD.—Cream butter and sugar; add Soyolk, and beat. Add beaten eggs. Beat in flour and milled walnuts. Beat the extra egg, stir in the chopped walnuts, add some to mixture. Put mixture in a greased tin, brush with egg. Pour over remainder of egg and walnuts to decorate. Bake in moderate oven for 1 hour (for shallow cake). Free edge of cake from tin before putting in oven—it gives room for expansion.

NUT CAKE

INGREDIENTS.—4 eggs, 6 ounces raw sugar, ¾ lb. milled nuts (Brazil, or hazel, or use 1 lb. walnuts).

METHOD.—Beat these and add 1 teaspoon baking powder. Bake in greased tin ¾ hour.

CARAMEL CAKE

INGREDIENTS.—1 cup raw sugar, 2 eggs, 2 teaspoons baking powder, pinch salt, ¼ lb. butter, 2 cups wholemeal flour, 1 teaspoon vanilla.

METHOD.—The day before making, put ¼ cup raw sugar in a small saucepan with 2 teaspoons water, and stir till sugar is melted, and the whole is a rich brown. Then pour ½ cup hot water over it. Cream butter and sugar, add egg yolks, flour and caramel alternately, and lastly fold in stiffly beaten whites. Bake in 2 tins.

TOPSY TURVY CAKE

INGREDIENTS.—1 egg, 1 cup wholemeal flour, 2 tablespoons butter, vanilla, 1 teacup sugar, 1 teaspoon baking powder, / cup milk or a little more.

METHOD.—Cream egg and sugar well, add melted butter and milk, flour, baking powder and essence. Give mixture a good beating. Melt 2 tablespoons butter in bottom of deep sandwich tin; spread evenly ½ teacup raw sugar, then ½ teacup chopped dates, and 1 teacup chopped walnuts. Pour cake mixture over the top of this, spread evenly and bake in moderate oven about 30 minutes.

ECONOMICAL WHOLEMEAL CAKE

INGREDIENTS.—1 tablespoon golden syrup, 1 cup cold water, ¼ lb. butter, ½ cup raw sugar, I cup raisins, 1 teaspoon each cinnamon and ginger.

METHOD.—Boil all ingredients together for 3 minutes. Stand aside to cool. Add 2 cups wholemeal flour, with 1 teaspoon baking soda sifted in. Bake for 1 hour.

SHORT CAKE

INGREDIENTS.—1 heaped breakfast cup wholemeal flour, 1 tablespoon raw sugar, 1 egg, 1 heaped teaspoon baking powder, ¼ lb. butter, a little milk.

METHOD.—Mix dry ingredients, rub in butter, mix with egg and milk. Roll and cut into squares. (This recipe may be used rolled thin for sweet pastries, such as dates, raisins, etc.)

ORANGE CAKE

INGREDIENTS.—¼ lb. each butter, raw sugar and flour, grated rind of orange, 1 teaspoon baking powder, 2 tablespoons coconut, 1 tablespoon orange juice, 2 eggs.

METHOD.—Cream butter and sugar, add egg, then flour and baking powder, coconut, orange rind and juice. Cook about 20 minutes.

COCONUT MERINGUE SHORTCAKE

INGREDIENTS.—1 cup wholemeal flour (fine), ¼ lb. raw sugar, 1 egg, ¼ lb. butter, 1 teaspoon baking powder, pinch salt.

METHOD.—Cream butter and sugar, add egg, then dry ingredients. Spread in bottom of greased tin. Cover with a little raspberry jam or marmalade.

Meringue: ½ breakfast cup raw sugar, 1½ cups coconut, 1 egg. Beat all together. Spread on top of jam. Bake in slow oven about 1 hour.

WHOLEMEAL CAKE (No Eggs)

INGREDIENTS.—4 cups wholemeal flour, 1 cup butter, ¼ teaspoon salt, 2 teaspoons cream of tartar, 1 cup raw sugar, 1 cup sultanas, 1½ cups milk, 1 teaspoon soda.

METHOD.—Mix in usual way, creaming butter and sugar, then adding other ingredients. Bake for about 1 hour.

ICED WHOLEMEAL CAKE

INGREDIENTS. — ¼ lb. butter, 3 tablespoons golden syrup, 1½ cups wholemeal flour, ½ cup chopped walnuts, ¾ lb. raw sugar, 2 eggs, 1 teaspoon spice, ½ teaspoon soda dissolved in ¼ cup milk.

METHOD. — Cream butter and sugar, add syrup and eggs, then dry ingredients, milk and soda last.

Icing: 1 cup raw sugar, 2 tablespoons butter, 2 tablespoons milk. Boil together for 2 minutes. Cook till thick.

SPONGE CAKE

INGREDIENTS. — 3 eggs, 3 tablespoons milk, 1 level breakfast cup wholemeal flour, 1 level teaspoon baking soda, 2 level teaspoons cream of tartar, small cup sugar, pinch salt, 2 tablespoons butter.

METHOD. — Beat eggs well, one at a time and adding the sugar gradually. Then add flour and baking soda, milk and butter melted together and lastly stir in cream of tartar. Hot oven 20 minutes.

BRAN CAKE DE LUXE

INGREDIENTS. — 4 ounces bran, 6 ounces each wholemeal flour, butter, seedless raisins, 2 ounces ground Barcelonas, 4 ounces candied peel, sour milk, 1 egg, ½ teaspoon cinnamon or spice.

METHOD. — Mix dry ingredients well. Add fruit and peel. Cream butter thoroughly. Beat the egg and add it gently to the butter. Sift in nuts. Melt treacle in some hot milk and cool by adding sour milk. Work butter into flour, bran, etc. Mix well and add treacle, etc., until mixture is creamy but not too wet. Place in rather shallow tins and bake in moderate oven 40 minutes. Leave in tin till cold.

CHESTER CAKE

INGREDIENTS.—6 ounces butter, 4 tablespoons raw sugar, 2 tablespoons cream of tartar, 2 heaped breakfast cups wholemeal flour, 2 eggs, 1 teaspoon soda.

METHOD.—Cream butter and sugar, add beaten eggs, then dry ingredients. Press half this mixture into large meat tin and cover with the following: Cut up dates, sultanas, raisins, spice, stale cake or biscuit crumbs mixed with water to moisten. Place other half of mixture on top, and cook in fairly quick oven.

NUTTIES

INGREDIENTS.—¼ lb. butter, ½ cup walnuts, 1 teaspoon baking powder, 1 small cup sugar, 1¾ cups wholemeal flour, 2 eggs, 1½ teaspoons spice, 1 cup dates.

METHOD.—Beat butter and sugar together; add eggs, then dates and walnuts; add dry ingredients. Place on cold buttered tray in spoonfuls and bake in fairly hot oven.

FRUIT SNAPS

INGREDIENTS.—3 cups wholemeal flour, ½ cup golden syrup, 1 teaspoon salt, 1 teaspoon spice, 1½ cups raw sugar, 1 cup raisins, 1 teaspoon ground cloves, 1 cup butter, 3 eggs, 1 teaspoon cinnamon.

METHOD.—Cream butter and sugar, add eggs singly, then syrup and fruit. Add flour, spices, and a teaspoon baking soda well sifted. Drop in teaspoonfuls on greased tray; flatten and put nut, cherry, or ginger on top. Bake in moderate oven 10 to 15 minutes. They keep quite well.

WALNUT BROWNIES

INGREDIENTS and METHOD.—Beat together ¼ lb. butter, and 1 teacup of sugar, add one egg and beat again. Mix together and add 1 breakfast cup of wholemeal flour, 4 teaspoons of cocoa, 1 teaspoon baking powder, ½ cup chopped walnuts. Roll out on greased tray and bake in moderate oven. Cut while warm and still on the tray.

WALNUT CRISPS

INGREDIENTS.—3 ounces butter, 3 ounces sugar, 6 ounces flour, 1 egg, 1 teaspoon ground ginger, ½ teaspoon baking powder, 2 tablespoons golden syrup, chopped nuts, essence to taste.

METHOD.—Cream the butter and sugar, add egg and dry ingredients as usual. Shape as a macaroon, decorate with halved walnut.

DATE CARAMEL CAKE

INGREDIENTS.—2 eggs, 1 cup raw sugar, 1½ cups dates, 3 cups wholemeal flour, 1 teaspoon vanilla essence, 2 tablespoons butter, 1½ teaspoons baking powder.

METHOD.—Cover dates with boiling water and stand for 3 hours or overnight. Beat sugar, eggs and butter; add dates, vanilla essence and flour. Bake 1½ hours in hot oven.

CHOCOLATE AFGHANS

INGREDIENTS.—6 ounces butter, 6 ounces flour, 1 tablespoon chocolate or cocoa, 2 ounces cornflakes, 3 ounces sugar, vanilla.

METHOD.—Cream butter and sugar; add dry ingredients, etc. Bake in moderate oven. Ice with a little chocolate icing and press on a ½ walnut.

LEMON DROP COOKIES

INGREDIENTS.—⅔ cup butter, 2 eggs, 4 tablespoons hot water, 1 cup sugar, ½ teaspoon soda, 1 tablespoon lemon juice, a heaped breakfast cup wholemeal flour, grated rind 1 lemon.

METHOD.—Cream butter and add sugar gradually; then eggs beaten till thick and light, then soda dissolved in hot water, lemon juice, rind and flour. Mix well. Drop from teaspoon on buttered baking sheet. Bake in quick oven.

CRUNCHIES

INGREDIENTS.—1 cup coconut, ¼ lb. butter, 1 cup sugar, 1 teaspoon soda, 1 cup wholemeal flour, 2 tablespoons hot water, 3 tablespoons treacle melted.

METHOD.—Put all dry ingredients in basin. Melt butter and add to melted treacle. Add soda and hot water and stir all into the dry ingredients. Mix well, roll into balls and flatten. Bake 10 minutes in a hot oven.

CHOICE CHRISTMAS CAKE

INGREDIENTS.—6 ounces wholemeal flour, 4 ounces sugar or honey, ½ lb. butter, 4 eggs, a little sour milk, 8 ounces ground almonds, 4 ounces ground walnuts, 1 lb. currants, 8 ounces seedless raisins, 6 ounces cherries, 6 ounces mixed peel, 1 teaspoon mixed spice.

METHOD.—Cream butter, add sugar and beat again. Beat eggs and add one by one to mixture of butter and sugar. Sift in dry ingredients and add fruit and peel. Mix with sour milk fairly moist. Put into greased tin and stand on 2 or 3 sandwich tins one above the other, having a thick layer of salt in the top one. Cook in slow oven 4 hours. Very slow the last hour.

LIGHT WHOLEMEAL CAKE

INGREDIENTS. — ¼ lb. butter, 3 eggs, 1 teaspoon cream of tartar, ½ cup milk, 1 cup raw sugar, 1½ cups wholemeal flour, ½ teaspoon soda.

METHOD. — Cream butter and sugar, add beaten eggs, then flour and cream of tartar, lastly soda dissolved in milk. Bake in meat tin in moderate oven.

LUNCH ROCK BUNS

INGREDIENTS. — 1 lb. flour, 1 cup milk, ½ lb. raw sugar, 1 cup mixed fruit, ¼ lb. butter, 1 teaspoon spice, 2 eggs, 1½ teaspoons baking powder.

METHOD. — Cream the butter and sugar. Add eggs well beaten and milk. Mix spice with the flour; add fruit and then the flour. Bake in spoonsful on oven tray or paper cases.

SHORTCAKE

INGREDIENTS and METHOD. — Cream ½ lb. butter with ¼ lb. raw sugar. With the hands work in 1 lb. wholemeal flour until dough is firm. Press into square tin which has been well greased. Prick well. Bake in very slow oven 1 hour. Cut into pieces before removing from tin.

ALMOND MACAROONS

INGREDIENTS. — ½ lb. butter, 1 level teaspoon baking powder, ½ lb. raw sugar, 1 egg, 13 to 14 ounces wholemeal flour, almond essence.

METHOD. — Cream butter and sugar, add egg and flour and baking powder and essence. Press an almond into top of small piece of mixture. Bake in moderate oven.

RAISIN MUNCHERS

INGREDIENTS.—2 ounces rolled oats, 8 ounces butter, 8 ounces sugar, 4 ounces coconut, 8 ounces wholemeal flour, 2 eggs, 2 tablespoons milk, ½ cup each raisins and almonds, juice ½ lemon.

METHOD.—Beat butter and sugar together to a cream, add eggs, then mix in dry ingredients. Break off small pieces a little larger than a walnut; place on cold slide and bake 15 minutes in moderate oven.

DATE SURPRISES

INGREDIENTS.—8 ounces wholemeal flour, 4 ounces butter, 3 tablespoons raw sugar, 1 egg, dates, nuts.

METHOD.—Cream butter and sugar, add beaten egg and flour. Roll out and cut into oblongs. Put a date stuffed with either a Brazil or walnut kernel on each oblong, fold over and bake.

WIGMORE CAKE

INGREDIENTS.—½ lb. of wholemeal flour, ½ lb. of sweet ground almonds, ½ lb. of butter, ¼ lb. of chopped citron, 1 lb. of currants, ¼ lb. of brown sugar, 1 whole nutmeg grated, 2 eggs, a little milk.

METHOD.—Mix dry ingredients thoroughly, melt fat and stir into the beaten eggs, add a little warm milk. Pour into dry ingredients and stir well. Make mixture moist but not too wet. Put into tin thickly lined with paper, stand tin on 2 or 3 sandwich tins to stop burning, cook in very slow oven 2½ to 3 hours. The success of this cake depends on the slow cooking and no other flavouring than the nutmeg.

PRUNE CAKE

INGREDIENTS. — 1½ breakfast cups wholemeal flour, 1 cup sugar, ¼ lb. butter, 3 eggs, 4 tablespoons prune juice, 1 teaspoon each cinnamon and spice, 1 breakfast cup cooked chopped prunes.

METHOD. — Cream butter and sugar, add eggs and beat thoroughly. Add flour and spices, then prune juice. Put prunes in last. Bake in moderate oven ¾ to 1 hour.

GOOD FRUIT CAKE

INGREDIENTS. — 1¼ lb. wholemeal flour, ½ lb. each butter, raisins, currants, ginger and chopped figs, 3 eggs, ¼ lb. peel, ¼ lb. raw sugar, 5 tablespoons black treacle, 1 cup sour milk.

METHOD. — Cream butter and sugar; add beaten eggs, flour and fruit. Warm the treacle and add; stir in milk and mix well. Bake slowly 2½ hours. Keep 14 days before using.

MADEIRA CAKE

INGREDIENTS. — ½ lb. of butter, ½ lb. of brown sugar, ¾ lb. of wholemeal flour, 2 eggs, 2 tablespoons of marmalade, ¼ lb. of walnuts if liked.

METHOD. — Cream butter and sugar, then add eggs and marmalade, then flour and 4. walnuts chopped up. Decorate top with the remainder. Bake 1½ to 2 hours.

PLAIN WHOLEMEAL RAISIN CAKE

INGREDIENTS. — 6 ounces of wholemeal flour, 4 ounces of butter, 4 ounces of seedless raisins, 1 egg, 1 tablespoon of brown sugar, 1 teaspoon ground cloves, 1 teaspoon of ground cinnamon, ½ teacup of sour milk.

METHOD.—Mix flour, cinnamon, cloves, sugar, and rub in fat, and add raisins. Beat egg, add sour milk and mix thoroughly with other ingredients. Moderate oven 40 to 50 minutes.

WHOLEMEAL SPONGE CAKE

INGREDIENTS and METHOD.—4 eggs, with their weight in butter, honey and fine wholemeal flour. Cream butter and work in honey; dredge in flour. Add eggs thoroughly beaten. Beat for 10 minutes at least, longer is better. Cook 20 minutes. When cool, but not cold, spread one half with sliced home candied peel, the other half with lemon or tangerine curd. Put together.

HONEY SHORT CAKE

INGREDIENTS.—4 ounces honey, 8 ounces butter, ¾ lb. wholemeal flour, 1 egg, grated rind 2 oranges.

METHOD.—Beat butter and honey to a cream; add the orange rind and flour. Mix with egg, using a little more flour if mixture is not firm enough. Roll out quickly and cut into squares. Place on floured trays and bake slowly 20 to 30 minutes.

ROLLED OATS SHORTBREAD

INGREDIENTS.—2 cups rolled oats, 1 cup raw sugar, 1 cup coconut, ¼ cup butter.

METHOD.—Place rolled oats, raw sugar, and coconut into a mixing bowl. Soften the butter and mix in with dry ingredients until the whole consistency is a crumbly mixture.

Grease a flat cake tin and press the mixture firmly into place. Bake in a moderate oven for 25 to 30 minutes. Becomes a golden brown and is crisp to eat. Keep in tin with Zwieback to keep hard. Cut in fingers for use.

PEANUT COOKIES

INGREDIENTS. — 1 breakfast cup wholemeal flour, 4 ounces butter, 1 teacup raw sugar, 1 egg, 1 cup shelled skinned peanuts, vanilla to flavour, 2 teaspoons cocoa.

METHOD. — Cream butter and sugar; add beaten egg. Stir in dry ingredients. Put in small lumps on a greased tray and bake 10 to 15 minutes in moderate oven.

WHOLEMEAL FRUIT CAKE

INGREDIENTS. — ½ lb. butter, 4 ounces sugar or honey, ¼ lb. walnuts, ¼ lb. mixed peel, 1 teaspoon mixed spice, ½ lb. wholemeal flour, 4 eggs, ¼ lb. almonds, 1 lb. each currants and raisins, ¼ lb. cherries, pinch salt, sour milk.

METHOD. — Cream butter and sugar, add eggs one by one, sift in dry ingredients, add fruit, nuts (chopped), and peel. Mix with sour milk to which has been added ½ teaspoon baking soda, make fairly moist. Put in greased tin and bake in slow oven with slide underneath for 4 hours.

TRILBY CAKES

INGREDIENTS. — 8 ounces fine wholemeal flour, 4 ounces butter, 4 ounces raw sugar, 2 teaspoons cinnamon, 1 teaspoon baking powder, ½ teaspoon baking soda, ¼ teaspoon salt, 1 egg, ½ cup chopped dates, ¼ cup each chopped walnuts and ginger.

METHOD. — Cream butter and sugar, add egg (a little milk may be used if necessary); add other ingredients and bake on cold greased trays 15 to 20 minutes.

CHEESE CAKES

INGREDIENTS and METHOD — Use recipe as above for pastry. Line patty pans with it and put 1 teaspoon raspberry jam at bottom of each. To this add the following mixture (about a teaspoon for each); Cream together 2 tablespoons butter and 2 of raw sugar, add 1 well beaten egg, sift in 3 tablespoons wholemeal flour and a little baking powder. Mix well.

Sandwiches

PASTES FOR SANDWICH FILLINGS

FRUIT PASTE: INGREDIENTS and METHOD.—Soak overnight some dates, figs and raisins in a small quantity of water. Mince and mix with half quantity minced apple, sprinkling cinnamon, dash of cloves.

EGG CREAM: INGREDIENTS and METHOD.—Lightly boil an egg, add finely chopped lettuce, chives and parsley, seasoning, mix well.

NUT PASTE: INGREDIENTS and METHOD.—1 ounce butter, 1 small teaspoon tomato paste, 1 dessertspoon Soyolk (Soya flour), 1 teaspoon Marmite, 2 ounces milled walnuts or almonds. Beat butter, Marmite and tomato paste, add Soyolk and mix well; then add nuts and pack into jars for future use.

MOCK CRAB: INGREDIENTS and METHOD.—2 ounces butter, ½ lb. skinned tomatoes, a little minced onion, 1 egg, 1 teacup bread crumbs, dash mace. Melt butter, add tomatoes, onion and mace and cook till soft. Beat well. Add eggs and breadcrumbs, and cook, stirring all the time. Pot and cover. (It will not keep very long.)

PLAIN BREAD AND BUTTER SANDWICHES

Use the following for fillings:—Thin slices of cucumber and grated radish. Seeded raisins and lettuce. Fruit paste. Egg cream. Mock crab paste. Nut paste. Savoury butter. Curried egg.

NOTE—Sometimes use sultana or raisin bread to vary these. (Fillings given in book.)

BISCUIT SANDWICHES

INGREDIENTS and METHOD.—Savoury cheese biscuits spread with milled nuts and cheese mixed to a paste and sprinkled with cinnamon.

Savoury cheese biscuits spread with grated raw carrot and cheese.

Weet-Bix, sliced, and covered with finely sliced figs, grated lemon peel.

CHEESE SANDWICHES (Various)

INGREDIENTS and METHOD.—Use wholemeal bread and butter for the base of these: grated cheese either plain or mixed with a little salad dressing and with one of the following mixtures:—Marmite, finely chopped spring onions, water cress; chopped parsley or sage; finely chopped dandelion leaves or spinach; finely chopped dates.

Beverages

WELSH NECTAR

INGREDIENTS and METHOD.—2 lb. raw sugar, 1½ packets seeded raisins, 4 lemons, 2 gallons water. Boil water and pour into large bowl to cool. Drop in the sugar. When quite cold add raisins and lemon rind, thinly pared, also juice. Stir and keep in cool place four days, stirring frequently. Strain through muslin and bottle. It is nice if kept 2 weeks before using.

[Note—we store our Welsh Nectar in robust swing top bottles and find that it is nicely fizzed after only a week. Keep an eye on the fermentation to avoid bottle explosions! Refrigeration will help to slow things down, S.A.H.B.]

CEREAL DRINKS
(To take the place of tea, coffee, and cocoa.)

There are several brands of cereal drinks on the market, but the two given here make a very good coffee substitute.

1. INGREDIENTS and METHOD.—Parsnips cut into thin rings, placed on oven tray and dried in oven until brown and crisp. Crush with rolling-pin and keep in air-tight tins. A little salt is an improvement.

2. INGREDIENTS and METHOD.—Four cups bran, 1 cup oatmeal, 1 cup golden syrup. Mix all ingredients, and bake brown in slow oven. Care must be taken that the cereal is thoroughly mixed with syrup. Use a deep baking tin and turn constantly while baking. Use 1 dessertspoon to each cup of water, simmer, strain and add hot milk.

LEMON DELIGHT

INGREDIENTS and METHOD.—4 or 5 sprigs fresh mint, 1½ lemons sliced very thin, 2 tablespoons raw sugar, ½ cup any fruit juice. Pour over all 1 quart of freshly boiling water. Serve cold.

GRAPEFRUIT AND APRICOT

INGREDIENTS and METHOD.— Wash and chop ½ lb. sun-dried apricots, soak in 1 pint water for 24 hours. Add more water if necessary to keep them covered. Strain through muslin and add juice of 1 grape-fruit. Sweeten with juice of soaked raisins or dates or honey. Dilute as desired.

About the Authors

Dr Ulric Williams (1890-1971) has been called 'New Zealand's Greatest Doctor' and yet the medical establishment made attempts to expel him from their ranks. Halfway through his career he rejected his surgical practices and allopathic prescriptions to become a naturopathic physician. Following an intensive period of reflection and scientific research he devised a complete outline of healthy living that cured patients through natural healing methods. As he once said, "I never became a real doctor until I forgot 95% of what I was taught at Edinburgh [Medical School]."

Dr Samantha Bailey trained and worked as a conventional doctor over two decades before a new understanding of health compelled her to leave the medical system. In 2020 she started what was to become New Zealand's largest Youtube health channel with her videos gaining millions of views and an international following. She is a co-author of *Virus Mania: How the Medical Industry Continually Invents Epidemics, Making Billion-Dollar Profits at Our Expense*. With her husband, Dr Mark Bailey, the couple have made their extensive collection of medical and health information freely available through their website www.drsambailey.com

Printed in Poland
by Amazon Fulfillment
Poland Sp. z o.o., Wrocław